T0290849

Testimonios of Care

Testimonios *of* Care

Feminist Latina/x and Chicana/x Perspectives on Caregiving Praxis

EDITED BY

NATALIA DEEB-SOSSA, YVETTE G. FLORES,

AND ANGIE CHABRAM

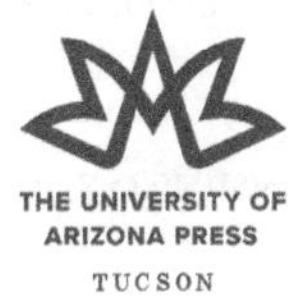

THE UNIVERSITY OF
ARIZONA PRESS
TUCSON

The University of Arizona Press
www.uapress.arizona.edu

We respectfully acknowledge the University of Arizona is on the land and territories of Indigenous peoples. Today, Arizona is home to twenty-two federally recognized tribes, with Tucson being home to the O'odham and the Yaqui. Committed to diversity and inclusion, the University strives to build sustainable relationships with sovereign Native Nations and Indigenous communities through education offerings, partnerships, and community service.

© 2024 by The Arizona Board of Regents
All rights reserved. Published 2024

ISBN-13: 978-0-8165-5322-8 (hardcover)
ISBN-13: 978-0-8165-5321-1 (paperback)
ISBN-13: 978-0-8165-5323-5 (ebook)

Cover design by Leigh McDonald
Cover art: *Virgen del Sol* by Alan Altamirano
Typeset by Sara Thaxton in 10/14 Warnock Pro with Electra LT Std

Publication of this book is made possible in part by the proceeds of a permanent endowment created with the assistance of a Challenge Grant from the National Endowment for the Humanities, a federal agency.

Library of Congress Cataloging-in-Publication Data
Names: Deeb-Sossa, Natalia, editor. | Flores, Yvette Gisele, editor. | Chabram-Dernersesian, Angie, editor.
Title: Testimonios of care : feminist Latina/x and Chicana/x perspectives on caregiving praxis / edited by Natalia Deeb-Sossa, Yvette G. Flores, and Angie Chabram.
Description: Tucson : University of Arizona Press, 2024. | Includes bibliographical references and index.
Identifiers: LCCN 2023048933 (print) | LCCN 2023048934 (ebook) | ISBN 9780816553228 (hardcover) | ISBN 9780816553211 (paperback) | ISBN 9780816553235 (ebook)
Subjects: LCSH: Women caregivers—United States. | Mexican American caregivers. | Hispanic American caregivers. | Hispanic American women. | Mexican American women.
Classification: LCC RA645.35 T47 2024 (print) | LCC RA645.35 (ebook) | DDC 362.14082—dc23/eng/20240321
LC record available at https://lccn.loc.gov/2023048933
LC ebook record available at https://lccn.loc.gov/2023048934

Printed in the United States of America
♾ This paper meets the requirements of ANSI/NISO Z39.48-1992 (Permanence of Paper).

Contents

Acknowledgments

This co-edited volume is the result of a long-standing femtorship, amistad, respect, and collaboration between Yvette G. Flores, Angie Chabram, and Natalia Deeb-Sossa. As colegas, we have supported each other's work and life projects. Our contributors' resistance and resilience inspired us. Our families, students, and community members accompanied us and supported our journeys as caregivers. Yvette G. Flores gives profound appreciation to Michele Ritterman, PhD, for all the years spent healing on her couch. Angie Chabram gives profound gratitude to Yolanda Butler for her care of Angie G. Chabram, her mother. Natalia Deeb-Sossa, in turn, gives heartfelt appreciation to Caleb Caudle for his years of feminist and equitable partnership. This book is in memory of Profesora Beatriz Pesquera, PhD.

Testimonios of Care

Introduction

ANGIE CHABRAM, NATALIA DEEB-SOSSA,
AND YVETTE G. FLORES

This book began through *pláticas* (heart-to-heart conversations) (Fierros and Delgado Bernal 2016; Flores and Morales 2021) in which we shared the courage it took to be women of color from different immigrant backgrounds in academia while becoming communal and familial caregivers. As *colegas*, friends, and mentors, our pláticas and *testimonios* facilitated presence, vulnerability, and self-reflection (Deeb-Sossa 2019; Latina Feminist Group 2001) on the authentic caring, or *cariño*, we were practicing every day with our partners, friends, mothers, or daughters. With open hearts, we listened to how our caregiving, or *cuidar*, included the work involved in navigating challenging social and physical ailments (Chabram-Dernersesian and de La Torre 2008; Facio 1995), relationships (Moraga 2019), structures, institutions, and borders. We knew we needed to document diverse caregiving experiences, as caregiving embodies the nature of the relationship (i.e., we care for a partner, mother/daughter, friend) and is also embodied in the praxis (i.e., how it is done; it is experiential). We also wanted to encourage others to share knowledge about caregiving that helps reveal how we live our cultural practices, our gendered norms, our rituals, and our *cuidado*, or care for one another. We also motivated others to take part in this volume in order to build solidarity and respond to and resist structures of oppression that promote invisibility and exclusion (Deeb-Sossa and Bickham-Mendez 2022).

In their testimonios, caregivers in this volume speak for themselves and document their own gendered relationships, cultural practices, and experiences, as both participants and witnesses in the systems of care. *Testimonios of Care* gives voice to those who often are voiceless in histories of caregiving. We hope this book will become a house of mirrors where diverse caregivers see themselves reflected, valued, and thus honored completely: body-mind-spirit (Lara 2002). We build on the legacy of the anthology produced by the Latina Feminist Group (2001), *Telling to Live: Latina Feminist Testimonios,* to inform our methodology. In this text, testimonios are theorized as "a form of expression that comes out of intense repression or struggle . . . an effort by the disenfranchised to assert themselves as political subjects through others, often outsiders, and in the process to emphasize particular aspects of their collective identity" (13). We also look to Gloria Anzaldúa's *Making Face, Making Soul / Haciendo caras: Creative and Critical Perspectives by Women of Color* (1990), which highlights how testimonio moves voices from the margins to the center and thereby "exposes brutality, disrupts silencing, and builds solidarity among women of color" (Delgado Bernal, Burciaga, and Flores Carmona 2012, 363).

The seeds for this volume are present in *Speaking from the Body* (Chabram-Dernersesian and de la Torre 2008), in which family members engage in care work, serve as advocates for family members and patients, and even tell the stories of those who cannot. To cite a few examples from the aforementioned volume, Yvette G. Flores memorializes her mother's struggles with dementia, providing an account and a voice that makes the testimony of this ailment possible; Citlali Sosa-Riddell and Bill Riddell intervene with their own personal caregiver observations in their mother's/wife's autobiographical depiction of Parkinson's; and Gabriela Arredondo's cancer narrative credits husband's and wife's efforts to participate in much-needed treatments in a timely way. In turn, Adela de la Torre documents the substantial changes experienced by her ailing mother (who suffers from rheumatoid arthritis) after she visits a psychologist, and Enriqueta Valdez-Curiel and Jessica Núñez de Ybarra fluctuate between their dual roles as doctors and daughters as they accompany their mothers; Dr. Núñez de Ybarra's testimonio describes her role as family member and consultant to her cousin as well. As physicians and family members, they help navigate their loved ones' healing journeys and administer different types of support. To further elaborate, *Speaking from the Body,* in which twelve Latinas voice how they deal with serious health episodes as patients, family caregivers, or friends, serves as a general source of inspiration in that those testimonios reveal how health status is shaped by gender, class, and race, and how family, spirituality, and culture can affect the experience of illness. These testimonios demonstrate how these health episodes shape every part of these Latinas' lives and how personal identity and community intersect to shape the interpretation of illness; compliance with treatment; and the utilization of allopathic medicine, alternative therapies, and traditional healing practices.

Furthermore, *Testimonios of Care* is guided by Chicana and Latina feminist principles, which include solidarity between women of color, empathy, willingness to challenge patriarchal medical health care systems, questioning traditional gender roles and idealization of *familia*, and caring for self while caring for loved ones and community. In the field of education, for example, Chicana/Latina scholars encourage us to draw upon cultural intuition (Delgado Bernal 1998). The roots of cultural intuition emerged from critical race feminist scholarship (Anzaldúa 2002; hooks 1989; Hurtado 1996; Walker 1982). Delgado Bernal (1998) described cultural intuition as "a complex process that is experiential, intuitive, historical, personal, collective, and dynamic" (567–68), highlighting how it is a process that embraces "one's personal experience to include collective experience and community memory" (563). According to Delgado Bernal, "cultural intuition" uses as sources personal experiences, collective experience, professional experiences, communal memory, existing literature, and the analytical research process (coding). Cultural intuition is constantly evolving and regularly becomes imbued with "spiritual activism"—"spirituality [that] can assist us in challenging racism, sexism, homophobia, and other forms of material psychic oppression" (Keating 2005, 243). While not included in the first description of cultural intuition (Delgado Bernal 1998), spirituality has been included for its significant role in nurturing this sight (Calderón et al. 2012). Thus, we "talk back" (hooks 1989) and "research back" (Smith 2021) against research methods and theoretical frameworks that are emblematic and support oppressive conditions and that reproduce deficit views about our communities. Given who we are and our experiences as caregivers, we use testimonios in this volume as a "pedagogical, methodological and activist approach to social justice" (Delgado Bernal, Burciaga, and Carmona 2012, 363) that engages with our collaborators in a critical meditation of their individual experience within discrete sociopolitical and economic materialities.

This co-edited book is the result of the vision, longtime collaboration, and friendship of the three co-editors, colegas who have spent years as caregivers for family members and partners as well as students. As we were working on this volume and carefully crafting this introduction, the world was rapidly changing around us with the rise of COVID-19, bringing new urgency to the topic of caregiving and foregrounding it as an essential practice and service of our time (Chatzidakis et al. 2020; Hobart and Kneese 2020).

Within the U.S. national context, news venues often reported that Latinas/os/xs[1] were an important part of caregiving, a fact that was made visible by the pandemic. The pandemic also drew attention to the multiple ways in which Latinas/Chicanas engaged in caregiving as they were strongly represented among the "essential workers" whose labor kept us fed as they toiled in fields, canneries, poultry factories, restaurants, and stores. They sustained and nourished all of us, and for those of us who had the luxury to work from home during the lockdown, they continued harvesting the food, driving the buses, cooking in the local restaurants, and cleaning our neighbors' houses. They enabled us to remain safe at home while many others risked their health and lives. This pandemic, as a result, dramatized the social, economic, and political disparities that affect Latina/o/x health and caregiving in a U.S. transnational context (Flores 2023).

However, our decision to refocus on Latina caregivers was not primarily a result of the pandemic or the fact the nation had become acutely aware of its dependency needs; rather, it emerged from a series of reflections regarding the historic importance of Latina care legacies in daily life, health, and culture and a lack of sustained critical attention to the multiple and dynamic forms of caregiving that have long existed among the Latina/o/x community amid many social crises and forms of dislocation. Together with other scholars, we contend that the spatial and conceptual separation between the public and private and the structural and ideological underpinnings of racialized social formations have contributed to the devaluing and marginalization of forms of caregiving intersected by race, class, gender, transnationality, sexuality, capitalism, and underpaid service work (see Nakago Glenn 2012).

Here we offer a correction to this state of affairs. We prioritize the communal right to tell and retell each caregiver's story and the right to be heard as individuals and as members of a writing collective and social group. We center the issue of what it is like to be a caregiver and how people produce meanings and practices out of diverse caregiver experiences and social po-

1. The term *Latinx* is used to contest the binaries and sexisms inherent in the Spanish language. However, we honor the authors' choice of terms in their essays.

sitions. Our work is thus fundamentally a work of representation as well as engagement and intervention. In our own rendition of caregiving, we prioritize our storied experiences, lived realities, and social practices and contexts (Nouwen 2011). We very intentionally highlight the Latinx caregiver and seek to restore a Latina feminist sensibility that inscribes Latina agencies, social imaginaries, and relational contexts, including those that are masculine. Following Suzanne Poirier and Lioness Ayres (2002), we believe that "the rich, detailed, contextual, and emotional nature of the stories bridge theory and practice" (xii). We find it useful to further clarify that we offer a partial representation—in daily life, Latinas/os/xs engage in monumental telling tasks, often in the presence of physical and emotional vulnerabilities, instances of pain suffering, worry, anguish—not to mention the structures imposed by racial, class, national, linguistic, educational, and gender privilege, all of which make the telling of something very difficult and burdensome. Yet despite these difficulties, Latinx caregiver expression continues to flourish in living rooms, neighborhoods, workplaces, community gatherings, and social relationships outside the home, wherever these caregivers converge. In this volume we capture a segment of this rich and bountiful expression, activating the notion of relationship building that has historically accompanied the *plática,* a historic form of moving into community from community.

This volume embodies the testimonios of diverse Latina/o/x caregivers in which each shares a snippet of their caregiving roles at a given moment in time. Each caregiver shares their experience, by employing testimonio, to challenge and contest the unvalued practice of caregiving that is seen as feminine and domestic labor. Centering their voices and stories challenges the invisibility, invalidation, and marginalization of the range of caregiving experiences. Therefore, we offer a breath and diversity of caregiving undertakings offered with sensibility and humility.

We view caregiving—cuidar, cariño—as authentic caring embodying the nature of the relationship (friend, partner, mother/daughter). It is also embodied in the praxis of how it is done every day in a material and experiential way. In these essays the Latinx caregivers describe their relational and embodied caregiving that is not just labor, not just transactional, but is an act of giving of themselves (ourselves).

We are giving care to a loved one, and this embodies, challenges, and reveals how we live our cultural practices; our gendered norms; our rituals; our cuidado, or care for one another. These testimonios of the practice of caregiving highlight how the act of caring is a relationship that binds the caregiver to their loved one more deeply through the witnessing of their health, illness, and pain. This caregiving relationship is complex and is shaped by the circumstances that each caregiver faces and the choices they can make. Here we celebrate one other's capability to care, underscoring how care receivers also reciprocate the care received, in their own unique ways. Everyone's caregiving is shaped by context, the nature of relationship, and mutuality/reciprocity.

So why this volume now? As caregivers, we wanted to give voice to our caregiving experiences. We also have been wounded in our relationships with the health care system as we, and our labor, have been treated and seen as disposable. We are wounded storytellers who believe that the act of telling and writing is healing. Finally, we hope that when we share these caregiving testimonios, readers will recognize themselves in them, and if so, that we can accompany them/you from afar in their/your caregiving journey.

In this volume, the first English-language collection of Latinx caregiving testimonios,[2] the expression covers multiple and diverse caregiving experiences that at times overlap and span a wide range of familial relationships, including daughter/mother (Enriqueta Valdez-Curiel, Angie Chabram), grandmother/grandson (yvonne hurtado allen), mother/son (Josie Méndez-Negrete), sister/brother (ire'ne lara silva), sister/sister (Anita Tijerina Revilla), aunt/nephew and aunt/niece (Anita Tijerina Revilla), and intimate co-care partnerships (Natalia Deeb-Sossa). In addition, the papers often register instances of self-care (Yvette G. Flores, yvonne hurtado allen), as well as caregiving situations that are rooted in professional relationships such as counseling (Yvette G. Flores, Hector Rivera-Lopez) and education (Natalia Deeb-Sossa, Mónica Torreiro-Casal). In addition, within this volume, caregiver situations are flexible, with doctors advocating for their mothers (Enriqueta Valdez-Curiel), daughters assuming caregiving roles for mothers (Angie Chabram) and siblings (Anita Tijerina Revilla), professors develop-

2. Other works inclusive of Latina caregiving practices generally span the fields of *curanderismo* studies (McNeill and Cervantes 2008; Perrone, Krueger, and Stockel 2012), the soldaderas of the Mexican Revolution, Latina healing (de Jesús Mosquera Saravia 2014) and psychology (Espin 1996), and issue-oriented accounts (Bruhn 2022; Nava-Schellinger 2021). In the Mexican context, Jonathan Yahalom's *Caring for the People of the Clouds: Aging and Dementia in Oaxaca* (2019) provides a regional Indigenous context.

ing community bonds that resemble familial ones (Mónica Torreiro-Casal, Natalia Deeb-Sossa), and caregivers developing strong intersubjective bonds of mutual intimacy and healing with care receivers across the board. Similarly, these caregiving situations cover a variety of ailments, including cancer, sexual abuse, trauma, chronic pain, inequality, underrepresentation, ageism, mental illness, substance abuse, and abandonment.

These caregiving narratives foreground the multiple roles and spaces the authors occupy. While offering care, the authors negotiate academic careers, often within heteropatriarchal and racist contexts; engage in social and political activism; participate in family life; and mentor and guide students and community members. Several of these authors lovingly provide care while facing health challenges of their own. Stories like these are rarely included in caregiving narratives written about caregivers who are women of color.

The authors' contributions offer examples of kinship care including formal and informal adoptions, community care, and caregiving in professional health contexts and visibilize the implicit caregiving inherent in teaching BIPOC students, which largely falls upon faculty of color, including Latinas/os/xs.

Although we understand that the knowledge base that is generated through these narrative acts is important to clinicians, doctors, and nurses, our motivation in producing this volume is not identical to books on narrative medicine that foreground the urgency of narrative competency among doctors and medical students. For us the goal is to engage in knowledge production that is generated by, for, and about the practitioners of Latina/o/x health. First and foremost, we hope to build and to publicize greater community-generated narrative competency among Latinas/os/xs with regard to these ailments, as a means to promote Latina health, wellness, empowerment, and self-determination.

Organization of the Book

The book is organized into three sections. Although several essays fall into multiple categories, we include narratives about kinship caregiving in the first section, including daughters caregiving for mothers/mother-in-laws (Enriqueta Valdez-Curiel, Angie Chabram, Anita Tijerina Revilla, Maria Angelina Soldatenko), mothers caring for their children (Josie Méndez-Negrete), the caring that emerges from informal adoption (yvonne hurtado allen, Anita Tijerina Revilla), sibling caregiving (ire'ne lara silva), and the caring that emerges in couple relationships (Natalia Deeb-Sossa).

The second section highlights community caregiving and care receiving in the context of authors' professional roles as psychologists (Yvette G. Flores, Hector Rivera-Lopez) and educators (Natalia Deeb-Sossa, Mónica Torreiro-Casal), as well as self-care (Maria R. Palacios).

The third section of our book offers the editors' final reflections as a call to action, as well as the Caregiver Bill of Rights, co-created by all the contributors to this book.

Intended Audience

Our book is intended for professional and lay audiences who will benefit from a more nuanced understanding of Latinx caregiving experiences. We intentionally invited artists and academics, community activists, and men and women to share their stories of providing care and to reflect on their experience through the lenses of their intersectional identities. We invited authors to consider their feminist ethics of care and the gendered nature of caregiving, as well as the ways in which cultural values, family context (social class, family economy, nativity, migration), birth order, gender, and family history of trauma impacted their lives and their caregiver role. We also invited their analysis, from their positionality, of the family legacies of caregiving.

Last, we invited their contributions to a Caregiver Bill of Rights that reflects the particularities of being a person of color—namely, a Latinx community member expected to adhere to cultural norms and caregiving patriarchal practices that may create stress. In this book we aimed to provide rich accounts of caregiving from a diverse group of Latinxs. We are of Caribbean, Central American, South American, Mexican, and Spanish origin. Some of us are immigrants, and some of us are descendants of original inhabitants of what is now the United States. Some of us are straight, and some of us are queer. Our identities and histories reflect the complex genealogies of peoples colonized by Europeans and impacted by diasporas. Inscribed in our bodies and spirits are legacies of trauma and survivorship. We offer these narratives as examples of resiliency.

References

Anzaldúa, Gloria E. 1990. *Making Face, Making Soul / Haciendo caras: Creative and Critical Perspectives of Feminists of Color.* San Francisco: Aunt Lute Books.

Anzaldúa, Gloria E. 2002. "Now Let Us Shift . . . the Path of Conocimiento . . . Inner Work, Public Acts." In *This Bridge We Call Home: Radical Visions for Transformation,* edited by Gloria Anzaldua and A. Keating, 530–38. New York: Routledge.

Bruhn, Sarah. 2022. "'Me cuesta mucho': Latina Immigrant Mothers Navigating Remote Learning and Caregiving During COVID-19." *Journal of Social Issues 79: 1035–56.*

Calderón, Dolores, Dolores Delgado Bernal, Veronica N. Velez, Lindsay Perez Huber, and Maria Malagon. 2012. "A Chicana Feminist Epistemology Revisited: Cultivating Ideas a Generation Later." *Harvard Educational Review* 82 (4): 513.

Chabram-Dernersesian, Angie, and Adela de la Torre, eds. 2008. *Speaking from the Body: Latinas on Health and Culture.* Tucson: University of Arizona Press.

Chatzidakis, Andreas, Jamie Hakim, Jo Litter, and Catherine Rottenberg. 2020. *The Care Manifesto: The Politics of Interdependence.* Brooklyn: Verso Books.

Deeb-Sossa, Natalia, ed. 2019. *Community-Based Participatory Research: Testimonios from Chicana/o Studies.* Tucson: University of Arizona Press.

Deeb-Sossa, Natalia, and Jennifer Bickham-Mendez, eds. 2022. *Latinx Belonging: Community Building and Resilience in the United States.* Tucson: University of Arizona Press.

de Jesús Mosquera Saravia, María Teresa. 2014. *Terapias ancestrales: Comadronas, curanderas y madres de familia.* London: Publicia.

Delgado Bernal, Dolores. 1998. "Using a Chicana Feminist Epistemology in Educational Research." *Harvard Educational Review* 68 (4): 555–82.

Delgado Bernal, Dolores, Rebeca Burciaga, and Judith Flores Carmona. 2012. "Chicana/Latina Testimonios: Mapping the Methodological, Pedagogical, and Political." *Equity and Excellence in Education* 45 (3): 363–72.

Espin, Olivia. M. 1996. *Latina Healers: Lives of Power and Tradition.* Encino, Calif.: Floricanto.

Facio, Elisa. 1995. *Understanding Older Chicanas: Sociological and Policy Perspectives.* Thousand Oaks, Calif.: SAGE Publications.

Fierros, Cindy O., and Dolores Delgado Bernal. 2016. "Vamos a platicar: The Contours of Pláticas as Chicana/Latina Feminist Methodology." *Chicana/Latina Studies* 15, no. 2 (Spring): 98–121.

Flores, Alma Itzé, and Socorro Morales. 2021. "A Chicana/Latina Feminist Methodology: Examining Pláticas in Educational Research." In *Handbook of Latinos and Education,* edited by Enrique G. Murillo, Jr., Dolores Delgado Bernal, Socorro Morales, Luis Urrieta, Jr., Eric Ruiz Bybee, Juan Sánchez Muñoz, Victor Sáenz, Daniel Villanueva, Margarita Machado-Casas, and Katherine Espinoza, 35–45. New York: Routledge.

Flores, Yvette G. 2023. "Mental Health During the Pandemic: Promoting Healthy Coping Strategies." In *Medical Humanities, Cultural Humility, and Social Justice*, edited by Dalia Magaña, Christina Lux, and Ignacio Lopez-Calvo, 155–76. San Francisco: University of California Health Humanities Press.

Hobart, Hi'ilei Julia Kawehipuaakahaopulani, and Tamara Kneese. 2020. "Radical Care: Survival Strategies for Uncertain Times." *Social Text* 38 (1): 1–16. https://doi.org/10.1215/01642472-7971067.

hooks, bell. 1989. *Talking Back: Thinking Feminist, Thinking Black*. Boston: South End.

Hurtado, Aida. 1996. *The Color of Privilege: Three Blasphemies on Race and Feminism*. Ann Arbor: University of Michigan Press.

Keating, AnaLouise, ed. 2005. *Entre mundos / Among Worlds: New Perspectives on Gloria Anzaldúa*. New York: Palgrave Macmillan.

Lara, Irene. 2002. "Healing Sueños for Academia." In *This Bridge We Call Home: Radical Visions for Transformation*, edited by Gloria Anzaldúa and AnaLouise Keating, 433–38. New York: Routledge.

Latina Feminist Group. 2001. *Telling to Live: Latina Feminist Testimonios*. Durham, N.C.: Duke University Press.

McNeill, Brian, and Joseph Michael Cervantes, eds. 2008. *Latina/o Healing Practices: Mestizo and Indigenous Perspectives*. New York: Routledge.

Moraga, Cherríe. 2019. *Native Country of the Heart: A Memoir*. New York: Farrar, Straus and Giroux.

Nakano Glenn, Evelyn. 2012. *Forced to Care: Coercion and Caregiving in America*. Boston: Harvard University Press.

Nava-Schellinger, Vivian. 2021. "Honoring the Stories of Hispanic Caregivers Unites Us All." National Council on Aging. Published October 5, 2021. https://www.ncoa.org/article/honoring-the-stories-of-hispanic-caregivers-unites-us-all.

Nouwen, Henri J. M. 2011. *A Spirituality of Caregiving:* The Henri Nouwen Spirituality Series. Saint Louis: Henri J. M. Nouwen Legacy Trust.

Perrone, Bobette, Victoria Krueger, and H. Henrietta Stockel. 2012. *Medicine Women, Curanderas, and Women Doctors*. Norman: University of Oklahoma Press.

Poirier, Suzanne, and Lioness Ayres. 2002. *Stories of Family Caregiving: Reconsiderations of Theory, Literature, and Life*. Indianapolis: Sigma Theta Tau International Nursing Publishing.

Smith, Linda Tuhiwai. 2021. *Decolonizing Methodologies: Research and Indigenous Peoples*. London, U.K.: Zed Books.

Walker, Alice. 1982. *The Color Purple*. New York: Harcourt Brace.

Yahalom, Jonathan. 2019. *Caring for the People of the Clouds: Aging and Dementia in Oaxaca*. Norman: University of Oklahoma Press.

PART I
The Caregiver Voice

CHAPTER 1

Scarred by the Medical Health Care System

Testimonio of Disappointment, Pain, and Transformation

NATALIA DEEB-SOSSA

Natalia Deeb-Sossa and her partner's entry provides an important illustration of co-caregiving. Here we see an important level of reciprocity that is often erased in representations of kinship arrangements. Also of importance is the role of advocacy in caregiving and the building of / being in a more equitable partnership. We see that these are very important components in situations where Western forms of diagnosis must be supplanted by the creative insights of *familias* who have to make healing from scratch in order for wellness to occur.

Introduction

This is a *testimonio* of friendship and love, of caregiving and hope, of pain and recovery, and of transformation and affirmation. Pain, because you feel powerless as your partner is in agony and depressed after more than eleven years in misery and six years out of work. Transformation, because in this arduous journey together, my partner and I had to reflect on how we connected, what we meant to one another, and how we supported, cared, loved, and empowered each other.

Our exploration was at times exciting and at other times exhilarating, but most of the time it was daunting. As a radical Xicana feminist, I always challenged myself politically and ideologically to not conform to stereotypical gender roles. I did not want to be recognized, affirmed, or validated by the cultural or social attributes that would supposedly make me a "good" woman or partner to a man.

Also, I had chosen my partner to be my life companion because he shared my politics and he embodied the elements that, I considered, made him a feminist partner. My partner continuously supports what is most important for me: community-responsive scholar activism in farmworker and immigrant communities, as well as teaching, scholarship, and engagement in the reproductive, immigrant rights, and feminist movements. Likewise, my partner is the person I go to first to ask for advice, to vent, and to cry (either because of joy or pain) due to my experiences in academia.

I approach the topic of caregiving for a male partner with our experiential knowledge and as our testimonio. We have experienced the effects of the for-profit health care system firsthand. Thus, I rely on our positionalities, unapologetically, to inform our critiques of the medical-industrial system as supported by research (Latina Feminist Group 2001) but also through my own experience as a caregiver.

Testimonios are "theory in the flesh" and embody the epistemologies of what is experienced through the body, mind, and spirit, as well as family, communities, and life experiences (Delgado Bernal, Burciaga, and Flores Carmona 2012).

My Partner

My partner was born in Santa Cruz, California, in 1969 to an unconventional single mother. He was enrolled in nine schools before eighth grade, as far east as Iowa and north as Canada, as his mother moved from relationship to relationship as a survival strategy.

After he obtained his GED, he grew up in the theater, the "first family [he] ever knew, and it was . . . very accepting."[1]

He then moved into a career in film and video, which he describes as "a little bit of rock and a little roll."

He was part of the lighting crew, the members of which, compared to the theater troupe, "had less neurosis, are less of a pretend artists, and are more real craftsmen."

1. All quotes in this chapter come from thousands of hours of *pláticas* with my partner during the years of co-caregiving. He has read the testimonio and given permission to quote him.

In video production, he concludes, "if you have integrity and the skill set, they are accepting; otherwise, you're shit out of luck." He liked going to work because every day the job was different, the crew was a tolerant family, and each person in the crew was accountable for their work.

When we met in 2009, animals and photography were shared interests. I had two cats and a dog, Thunder, whom I took everywhere. I also loved taking portraits of people. He, on the other hand, had just lost his two lifelong dog companions of fifteen years, Jeb and Bundy, and did wildlife photography.

When I asked how he got into wildlife photography, he said this:

> Photography has always been in my background. Mostly because my mother was interested in it and had her own stint at pretending to be a great photographer. I bought my first camera while working in theater. I had a friend who worked in a local camera store who gave me a discount, and I bought a professional-grade camera. I was young and never really learned to use it. I was always into backpacking, and so I rearranged my gear in order to carry as much as I could and to capture whatever I could. I was just taking pictures, never figuring out what it was that I was trying to capture, just snapping pictures but never had an agenda about it. I hadn't figured out the thing I like to take. Until I stumbled across a fawn that I spooked his mother away, frozen in the brush, and I snapped a picture of it. That's what gave me the bug. It was in the nineties, in Cedar or Desolation, miles out there.

He traveled thousands of miles to get away from work, from technology and humanity:

> I drove until there was no internet signal and then some. At the beginning it was mostly just a thing to do. Backpacking with the dogs, dragging my camera around, and I would get pictures of the dogs, of scenery, or of wildlife.

One of his fondest memories "out there" occurred in Sheldon, Nevada, far off in a dirt road: "I found a great horned owl's nest, and a hundred feet from it, in another tree, a red-tailed hawk's nest. I gave it everything I could while I was there. I continued to go back to that same spot for three years. Every time I went by there, I checked if there was anybody in that nest."

But as Joan Holloway from *Mad Men* noted, "One minute you're on top of the world. The next minute, some[one] is running you over with a lawnmower."

Series of Unfortunate Events

Our downfall was an accident and a series of very unfortunate events at the hands of incompetent health care providers.

He spent a week in and out of a photo blind and sneaking out in the middle of the night trying to photograph a red-tailed hawk on a nest. He, six feet tall, ended up as a pretzel in a four-by-four blind sixteen hours a day. He tried several times at the same spot, trying to get the photo. Between attempts, he drove home because he had to work, but right after work, he would drive back out, nine hours, to that same spot and sit in the blind for three or four days straight and get up the next morning and drive nine hours home and work the next day.

Then everything changed. He recalls:

> I was rotating the truck's tires because I had put so many miles on, and that's one thing I learned is that I needed to keep the truck maintained because I was so far out there. I did all of the work on the truck, as it allowed me to afford camera gear. Doing as much stuff as I could on my own when I could. So, as I was changing a tire, sure enough, it just managed to slip. I was on the floor for twenty minutes. I couldn't move and immediately went to the doctor the next day.

He went to Kaiser, and his primary doctor at the time ordered some x-rays and sent him home to rest from a so-called back strain. Being an independent contractor, he could take weeks off and recoup.

However, the reality was that he needed to go to work after a month of recuperation. In 2009, after a month or two of working full time as a member of the lighting crew, he injured himself again.

Somewhere in the South Bay, early one morning, they were shooting an exterior of a building. The lighting crew had set up a track and a dolly, and they were waiting for production to roll up so they could "push the button," or start recording, as the sun was rising, in order to get all the magic light

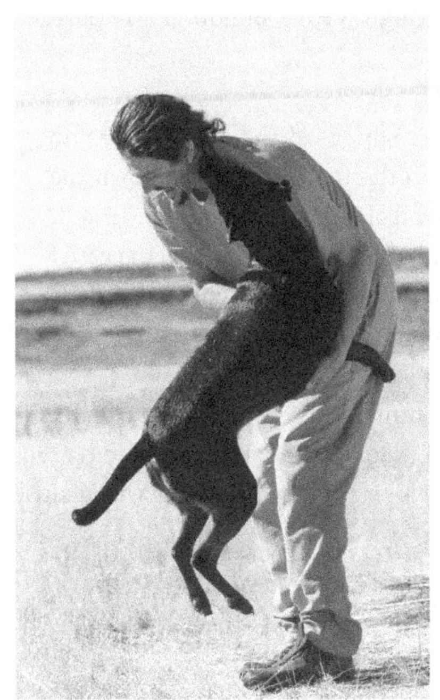
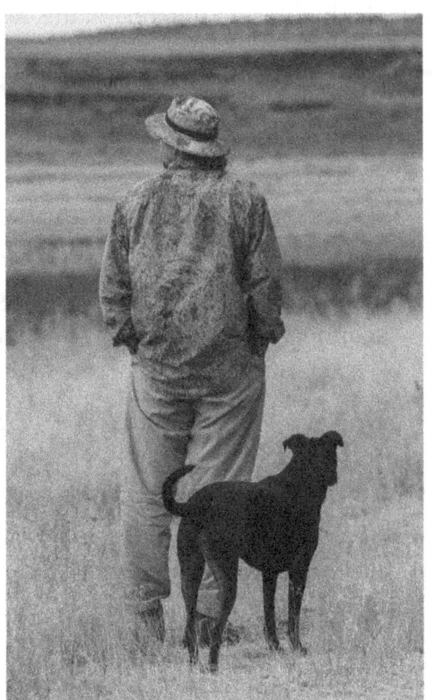
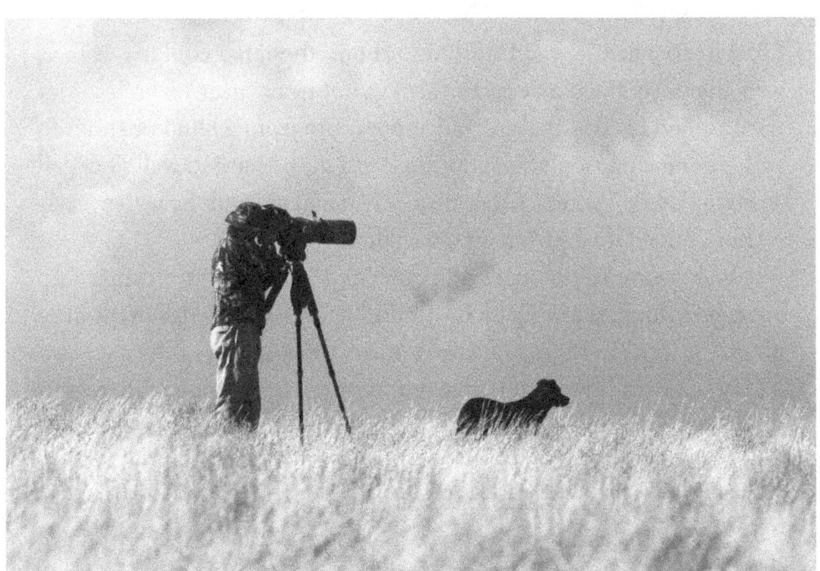

FIGURE 1.1 My partner and Thunder.

on the building. Someone came, shouting "Wrong building." My partner recalls,

> We're a block away from where we're supposed to be. There was no time to break the gear down, put it in the truck, and drive down the block. We had to pick up the dolly on the track and double-time it down the street. Whatever recuperation I had gained and all the care I had given myself after weeks and weeks I took off went out the window. I completely blew it out right then and there.

My partner immediately made an appointment to see his primary doctor in Kaiser. At the appointment, he insisted, "Hey, there's something going on." However, the doctor persisted, saying, "Nope, don't see anything wrong. Just take it easy."

As per doctor's instructions, he took more time off, rested, and tried to do all the right kinds of exercises. Since nothing was "wrong" after six months of rest, he tried to get out to the wild, hike, and take photographs. He recollects,

> I had to change the way I started to shoot, though. I couldn't walk as well anymore. I couldn't carry this kind of heavy gear for miles. So I tried to find critters that I could shoot more from a blind or shoot in and around a particular location so that I didn't have to walk. I began sneaking up on critters. Close distance in and around the water.
>
> But I ended up injuring myself again.
>
> I was trying to do an army crawl, and I had to lift a camera up over something, sneaking up on sandhill cranes at the edge of the little pond. I just made a move, a wrong move, the slightest of things.
>
> My back was always hurting, and it never has stopped. There was a weakness already; there was something. It was set up to fail at some point. It was inevitable!
>
> That third injury, that third time, I heard the loudest pop I have ever heard come out of my body. It was the most excruciating pain I have ever had . . .
>
> I don't know how it happened and how I could've done that in such a maneuver . . .

> I lay there for an hour or two before I could literally drag myself back to the truck. I sat a day or more in the camper, not being able to drive out.
>
> Then I drove eleven hours at least. I went straight to the doctor the next day.
>
> Any guesses on what he said? "Nothing on the x-rays. Get some rest."

But despite the rest, his damaged body was not willing to suppress the pain and the wounds and refused to keep silent.

As his partner, I struggled to support him, to maintain my sanity, and to bear witness to his pain.

Drug Pushers

My partner has lived (managed, survived) for eleven years (and counting) with intense chronic pain. The doctors at Kaiser, despite not finding the cause of the pain, ran him through a number of drugs, none of which even touched the pain. However, as he recalls, most of them were just "brewing in my gut ever so. I went in there twice, three times a year complaining of exactly the same thing, and I was continually just shrugged off. That went on for four years at Kaiser. As far as they could tell me, I just work too hard. I play too hard. I can't shake this. So I thought it must be some sort of strain that I continually reinjured. I had zero advice from Kaiser, zero help."

When I asked what kind of medicine they gave him at Kaiser, he mentioned opioids and prednisone.

Prednisone is a synthetic steroid given orally for inflammation. This synthetic mimics the action of cortisol (hydrocortisone)—the naturally occurring corticosteroid produced in the body by the adrenal glands.

When on prednisone, as on any steroid, his metabolism ramped up and he felt enraged. He also could not fall asleep at night. He noted,

> I was cranked up. I hated it. It turns out that anything that might even corral the pain only makes it worse.
>
> Imagine you've got a broken leg and they give you something so you can't feel the leg. That doesn't make the leg any better; it just means

you're going to walk around on it. It's going to hurt more when that drug wears off.

It's just really what happened.

I mean, when the drug wore off, I felt worse than when I started because it gave me the ability to be up. So, yeah, I hated it, and I said I'd never do that again, and shortly thereafter, I blew a fuse. First time in my life, I went home in the middle of a day's work.

I asked him, "What do you mean, you blew a fuse?"

I thought I was stressed more than I was hurting. I couldn't really tell. I couldn't tell what was bothering me more, the stress of life or the amount of work. That day, I was breaking out into sweats.

In the first couple of locations, I'm just hopping all over the place.

We're working at some hospital, ironically. We found ourselves in the hospital, interviewing nurses or doctors. We're walking down the hall and rolling stuff around, and everybody would look at me. Every nurse that passed me had to stop me and say, "Are you okay?" and I'm just like, "I don't know, I'm working. I'm just trying to work."

I was sweating and just boiled over. Some nurse pulled me aside when we had finally set up and I could rest a little bit: "Maybe you just need some sugar?" "I'll give you some hospital orange juice." "Little hospital milk."

We wrapped that location and packed everything up and drove off to lunch at the next location. I just started to hurl. My boss at the time said, "Why don't I just take you home?"

I just gave in. "Yeah, I think that's probably best."

I've called in sick, called in sick on work, maybe once, but a day or two ahead of time, and I might've been ten or fifteen minutes late somewhere towards the end of my career here and there, and it was routine jobs. This was a first!

When my partner's body "boiled over," it was his body rejecting all the narcotics and steroids that were masking the pain. The narcotics and steroids only masked the illness and did not heal his body. As my partner lay in the emergency room, giving voice to the atrocities committed in the name of medicine, and as he named the traumatic events that marked his body, he reclaimed some power around his healing.

Doctors use their power, authority, and knowledge over their patients and determine the course of people's recovery or management of pain.

From then on, I went with my partner to all his doctors' appointments, not as a detached observer but with loving and caring enthusiasm.

Disability, Obamacare, and Management of Pain

The reality was that my partner could not return to work. He physically would not be able to do the job. It demanded, for example, being on his feet for more than three or four hours and going up and down ladders carrying fifty to one hundred pounds of lights or other gear.

This meant that as an independent contractor, he kept his health insurance with Kaiser as long as he could afford it. But that only lasted a year.

Meanwhile, he did all the paperwork and applied for the Affordable Care Act, or Obamacare. Once he was accepted at a local community clinic, he had to wait almost eleven months to see his first primary care provider.

Not surprisingly, health care is not always equitable. Unfortunately, the first primary health care provider "was a snob" (i.e., a young white male), and my partner asked to be seen by another provider (female).

In this community clinic, as in Kaiser, the primary health care providers were ill equipped to care for his complex case. My partner's pain always manifested in the lower back, but he had a hip problem.

Despite his self-advocacy and insistence that they look further to find the underlying problem, they missed the diagnosis. It took five years, two other health care systems, and more than a handful of specialists (i.e., pain management specialists, physical therapists, orthopedists, a back surgeon, and a neurosurgeon) before my partner got diagnosed with a labral tear in the left hip and avascular necrosis (AVN).

A hip labral tear affects the labrum, or the ring of cartilage that follows the outside rim of the socket of the hip joint. When undamaged, the labrum cushions the hip joint and acts like a rubber seal or gasket to help hold the ball at the top of the thigh bone securely within the hip socket.

AVN is the death of bone tissue due to a lack of blood supply. AVN can lead to tiny breaks in the bone and the bone's eventual collapse. In my partner's case, the use of prednisone, a high-dose steroid medication, is believed to have interrupted the blood flow to the bone. His provider in Kaiser was the one who prescribed prednisone.

WTF! . . .

This is a clear example of what Dr. Armando Morales (1972) in *Ando sangrando* introduced as the medical term *iatrogenic*, which Roberto Cintli Rodriguez, in *Yolqui, a Warrior Summoned from the Spirit World: Testimonios on Violence* (2019, 64), described as "the American iatrogenic solution," explaining,

> Iatrogenic is primarily a medical term to denote that a problem, condition or disorder is induced, produced or aggravated by the physician or healer. In other words the healer makes the problem worse.

When we learned that something a doctor prescribed had caused the AVN, we felt indignant and disappointed.

Surgery and Potential Transformation

After living with chronic pain for approximately eleven years, having a diagnosis suggested we could come up with potential solutions.

But why did the potential solution come so late? One reason was that my partner's injury had a very asymptomatic presentation. He did not present like 90 percent of patients with the same injury. Health care providers are trained to consider characteristic expressions of illnesses. Therefore, when my partner was insisting that it hurt in the back and not in the front, they ignored his pain and even implied at one point that it was all in his head.

No health care provider has been able, after eleven years, to explain his spasms. As he describes,

> Nobody [no doctor or specialist] will try to connect those dots . . . Zero interpretations, speculation, or idea of what the spasms are or how the physiology is working. Why it hurts where it hurts and why it doesn't hurt where it's supposed to. Even he [an orthopedic surgeon] just wouldn't even speculate and you bring it up to half of any of them.

> They don't even want to see it. They're like, you bring it up, and they're like, they change the fucking subject because that is something they don't want to be liable for. They can't. It's out of their box. They can't say anything about it. They can't offer any explanation as to the root of the pain because it's out of their box, and if they say anything about it, that makes them then responsible.

Despite the trauma and the little faith we had in the health care system, we decided to follow the orthopedic surgeon's recommendation. The surgeon recommended that my partner have a left hip arthroscopy, labral repair, femoral head recontouring, capsular repair, core decompression, and autologous bone marrow nucleated cell transplant to femoral head.

This meant that my partner's bone marrow was collected, then sent to be processed, or spun down using a centrifuge. This created a concentrated sample of stem cells. While the bone marrow was being processed, the surgeon was performing the hip arthroscopy. The six-hour surgery ended after the stem cells were injected while the open core decompression was performed.

But what is next?

He is now over ten years older than when he was injured, and as he describes it, he is now "broken," "patched," but "not repaired." Therefore, for us, "there is no getting back to where [he] was. There's some other life."

When we try talking about it, he does not want to discuss it:

> I don't know. I don't even want to think about it . . . No. It's absolutely demoralizing. I've tried so many times to try to reinvent my future in my head and focus myself in the shop, to focus myself in the wild. As a physical person, I don't have faith in that, whatever that is. It won't be anything like what I was able to do because I'm ten years older, but it's like thirty years older, physically.

It is very hard, as a partner, to see the person you love be in chronic pain, have sleepless nights, suffer from rage and anger due to steroids and depression, and wonder how much that is taking a toll on his life expectancy.

I have been by my partner's side since July 2009, witnessing how he has been going through eleven years of agony. How do you convince him that all his potential has not "turned to dust," as he often mentions to me when we are talking about our future?

Caregiving and Despair

As caregivers, we are completely unprepared to support our loved ones when they are suffering chronic pain and suicidal ideation.

As I understand it, chronic pain is a medical condition in which our loved one is suffering from constant pain, and this debilitating condition does not allow them to enjoy life to the fullest, as it limits what they can do. It is not surprising, then, that our loved one who suffers from chronic pain is over five times more likely than acute pain sufferers to express a desire to die because of pain. The role of perceived burdensomeness is an important factor in suicidality (Kwon and Lee 2023). Perceived burdensomeness is the belief that one is a burden to others, does not contribute, and is a liability to the well-being or safety of others.

Pain-related factors of suicidality for our loved one with chronic pain are depression, disability, sleep problems, and hopelessness, to mention a few.

So how do we support, assess, and intervene when suicidality is such a stigmatized and sensitive topic among family, loved ones, and caregivers?

How, as caregivers, do we identify suicidality risk factors and harmful risk factors and discuss them openly with our loved one and suggest they see someone?

How do caregivers try to not succumb to the worry of not doing enough, of not loving enough, of not caring enough, of not saying "*Te amo*" enough?

The scariest part for my partner and for me is that we don't really seem to have any choice in what the future brings. We don't know what we would have chosen to do differently. But what is next?

After giving up his career, his identity, and his friendships, is going back to "normal" good enough?

According to my partner, quoting one of his favorite movies, *Buckaroo Banzai*, "No matter where you go, there you are." He explains,

> When you don't have any control, you make do with what you have, and you make do with where you end up. I'm going to make the best of it, with the same integrity to life and commitment. Not being com-

placent, of course. I need to remind myself, this is really great. What can we do with this?

Together we will continue to support each other in our journeys and through our challenges. Every day I am reminded of why I fell in love with him: due to his integrity, his relentlessness, his self-determination, and his *ganas.*

Collaborative Caregiving

Unfortunately, a lifetime in academia, as well as *susto, angustia,* and feeling helpless, took a toll on my health, and I began to suffer generalized anxiety, migraines with aura, and irritable bowel syndrome.

In 2021 I ended up having surgery for a paraesophageal hiatal hernia, as part of my stomach was protruding up through an opening in the diaphragm, and as a result I was experiencing gastroesophageal reflux disease. My partner nursed me back to health and accompanied me to my telehealth appointments. He now advocated for my health and recuperation.

Lessons

He has always been a private person, but he knows how important it is for me to teach and for others to learn from our experiences. What are the lessons here?

Advocate for yourself and loved ones. If you are not satisfied with what your doctor is telling you, seek a second, third, fourth, and fifth opinion.

Equity in health care is important. The health care insurance that you can purchase should not determine the quality of your care.

We offer our testimonios as a means for collective survival. Testimonios give life to collective experiences of scarring by the medical system, of pain at the hands of medical doctors, but also of transformation, while unapologetically responding to issues of health care inequity and resisting health care policies that perpetuate inequities.

Through testimonios on caregiving we might gain greater insight on how the medical-industrial complex impacts Chicana and Latina caregivers. Testimonios might help us understand the many implications of the current medical health care system on caregivers who are women of color. Shared testimonios may be crucial to understanding collective survival and solidarity across communities of women of color.

References

Delgado Bernal, Dolores, Rebeca Burciaga, and Judith Flores Carmona. 2012. "Chicana/Latina Testimonios: Mapping the Methodological, Pedagogical, and Political." *Equity and Excellence in Education* 45 (3): 363–72.

Kwon, Chan-Young, and Boram Lee. 2023. "Prevalence of Suicidal Behavior in Patients with Chronic Pain: A Systematic Review and Meta-analysis of Observational Studies." Frontiers in Psychology 14. https://doi.org/10.3389/fpsyg.2023.1217299.

Latina Feminist Group. 2001. *Telling to Live: Latina Feminist Testimonios.* Durham, N.C.: Duke University Press.

Morales, Armando. 1972. *Ando sangrando (I Am Bleeding): A Study of Mexican American-Police Conflict.* La Puente, Calif.: Perspectiva.

Rodríguez, Roberto Cintli. 2019. *Yolqui, a Warrior Summoned from the Spirit World: Testimonios on Violence.* Tucson: University of Arizona Press.

CHAPTER 2

Perfect Moments

On the Intersection of Being a Chicana with Diabetes and My Brother's Caregiver

IRE'NE LARA SILVA

ire'ne lara silva's piece offers a detailed and complex description of care work. Here, care work is intentional, multirelational, familial, and intersectional. Sister and brother care for one another, although the sister is the primary caregiver as well as the one who must administer the bulk of her own self-care. Aside from providing a list of tasks that must be done, she is also employed, and this job again and again struggles to negotiate and value the care role. While medical establishments are repeatedly ignorant of the multiple forms of caregiving that require support, this essay highlights them in describing the intimate bonds that unite brother and sister and make successful care and health outcomes possible.

It wasn't a perfect day. It was a perfect few hours. First Saturday of November in Austin. Sunny and warm enough for shorts and sandals. A generous wind rippling through grass and trees, singing into our hair and against our faces. It had been a few years since we'd made it to the annual Austin powwow, an all-day event organized by the nonprofit organization Great Promise for American Indians.

We spent those perfect hours listening to the drum circles and the singing, watching the dancers, eating fry bread and roasted corn, and winding our way through the vendors' stalls, where my brother found three turtles—one ceramic, one wooden, one stone—that had to come home with us. I pushed his wheelchair this way and that, around the stadium seating, up and down inclines, onto and off the grass. At the end of the day, a young man working the door generously gave up his plastic folding chair so I could sit while we waited for the paratransit bus to pick us up and take us home.

We were both content, if a little achy. It'd been a long day. The perfect hours had been preceded by our getting up early to have breakfast and take medications, by my helping him with an in-bed bath, by three hours of waiting, by my throwing a fit over an uncooperative paratransit bus driver, and then by a solid hour of insisting on our right to prompt transportation with person after person on the phone. I'd scheduled a pickup for 10:00 a.m., but we didn't leave for the powwow till almost 1:00 p.m. I refused to give up. I was angry at the unfairness of it all, but mostly because although my brother didn't say anything, I could see how he was folding in on himself with disappointment. The powwow was part of our weekend celebrating his birthday. Also, although there are days when I am battling overwhelm and exhaustion, I can also become the most stubborn person I have ever known. I pushed and pushed until a new bus came, picked us up, and drove us across the city.

It was dark already when we got home. Both of us were exhausted. I was stumbling while I made sure he was comfy in bed, then pushed his wheelchair out of the way, brought him fresh water, left a snack in case he woke up and needed one, and made sure that his pain medication, his phone, and a portable urinal were within his reach. And then we both fell asleep for four hours and were starving for dinner when we woke up.

This is often what life feels like. Working like hell to prepare everything, troubleshooting chaos, drinking in the sweetness of living as it comes, struggling to do all the things we should do, and then falling down exhausted.

I wish I could say that I am on top of everything. That all our meals are organic and 100 percent diabetic friendly and full of protein. That we eat every day on a regular schedule. That I pack all my lunches and snacks at the start of every week. That I am on top of every medication we both take—calling refills in to the pharmacy well in advance, reapplying to patient assistance programs as needed, restocking both our weekly pill containers before they run out—and that we both manage to take all our medication on schedule. That we both make it to all our doctors' and specialists' appointments and never have to reschedule, never forget an appointment, never feel too bad or too tired to see a doctor. That our lab work always reflects perfect numbers, or at least ever-improving numbers. That they never fluctuate wildly, that they obey our wishes, that they tell the story of how hard we try.

Sixteen years into supporting us both, and with his most recent disability application still pending, I wish I could say that making co-pays and keeping up with things like a new manual wheelchair are never a problem. I wish I could say that our apartment is always perfectly clean, the laundry done, the fridge stocked, the plants watered. I wish I could afford a home health aide and a physical therapist for him on my salary. I wish my workdays didn't require me to be gone for almost twelve hours every day. I wish I could work from home but keep my job—only five years left till retirement, after all. I wish I could say that I have organized calendars and a system of automated alerts for every facet of our lives. I wish I could say that I've figured out how to take care of him and how to take care of me and that these two priorities never have a conflict. That I don't sometimes—every day, or, more honestly, every hour—have to choose and choose and choose again, solving for some magical unknown balance. Always asking, What's the priority right now?

There's always work. For twenty years I've worked a full-time job as an administrative worker, first for the State of Texas and then for the County of Travis. Most of those years, I also worked a part-time job—doing a multitude of things, including retail work, housekeeping, caregiving, driving, mail clerking, and working for a literary arts organization. Some of those years I worked the additional job from home, but most of them were spent outside the home, which meant very long hours away. It's only been since February of 2018 that I was able to work just the one full-time job. Of course, this doesn't include my freelance editing/consulting work, writing, or speaking gigs—commitments that have steadily grown in the last decade.

That's the other major part of the equation—the writing, and the writing career. In the years before my first book and for some time after, I knew the writing hardly made sense to anybody. It seemed eminently more sensible to expend that time, energy, and visualization on other things. It made more sense to do anything else—to spend my resources on taking better care of myself and my brother, to spend them on getting promoted at work in the hopes of a raise, to spend them on going back to finish my degree, or even to spend them on rest and sleep and bingeing Netflix.

But writing is what makes everything make sense. Writing, my writing community, organizing literary events, and dreaming my books and writing life into being were what sustained me before, during, and after the years of relentless struggling. Writing is what made and what makes the daily calculations, the endless juggling, and the frustrations bearable. Beyond caring for myself and for my brother, writing is what gives my life purpose. And it was writing that allowed me to make my peace with diabetes.

I was diagnosed as diabetic and started on insulin on April 23, 2008. I was thirty-three years old. The first four years were filled with crushing fear, a constant overwhelm that darkened my days and left me reeling. I did what my doctors told me, I took care of my brother, and I worked sixty-plus hours a week in order to keep a roof over our heads and food on the table. At first, I lost weight, and then I regained it all and more besides. More medications. More insulin. The pain in my body became more incapacitating, but there was no choice but to keep on going.

In the fourth year of being diabetic, I started writing poems about diabetes. I wrote what I couldn't find. I started *Blood Sugar Canto* with the intention of writing about my experience of diabetes. And not just mine, but my family's, my communities'—and every way in which it seemed that a chronic illness could impact a life. That is to say, it impacts every part of life.

I wrote *Blood Sugar Canto* because I wanted to move past my fear. There was no way I could understand fear as being part of the way to heal. No way I could understand fear as helping me to take care of myself. But it seemed like everything in Western medicine was based on fear—making people afraid so that they obeyed doctors without questioning and took whatever pills were prescribed to them. Fear and shame were what doctors used to make their patients obey and change their diets and start exercising.

In every way, I cried out against fear being what set the parameters of my life. I wanted love to be what drove me to care for myself and others, love to be what lent me wisdom and understanding, love to be what informed me of what my body/heart/spirit/mind needed in order to be healthy and strong.

In the process of writing the poems for *Blood Sugar Canto* and in the process of figuring out how to restructure our lives after my brother's diagnosis in 2005 and mine in 2008, it became clear that there were many beliefs that needed questioning.

We hear a lot about self-care, but the way I grew up, taking care of others was sacred and honorable work. Taking care of yourself was selfishness and arrogance. It was to put yourself above others—your community, your parents, your children, your loved ones. It was to refuse to be of service, and there were hardly worse possible things for a woman to do. Others could demand what they needed—but a woman's first and last thought each day was supposed to be for others. Even prayers were prayed on behalf of others, not for oneself.

But living with diabetes demands a foundational shift in this way of thinking. In no way am I a model of self-care or of putting myself first. Even after eleven years of living with diabetes, I am often stretched way too thin and am still likely to put almost everything ahead of myself. But as much as I've pushed forward on willpower alone, it's also true that my experience of diabetes has included what I call "the wall"—the point at which my body just refuses to go on, no matter what I tell it, no matter what I will, no matter what is needed. Over time, I've had to learn to listen to my body, to realize that for myself, for the caregiving, and for my writing, I have to give my body what it needs and wants. And that I have to prioritize this giving to myself. Otherwise nothing else is possible.

I also think that there's a fundamental difference in the understanding of what a body is and what it's for. At first I thought it was a cultural difference between attitudes prevalent in Western medicine and attitudes prevalent among people of color. But upon more reflection, I think it's actually a class difference between working-class/poor people and middle-class/affluent people. Among the working-class/poor people I grew up with, a body's principal purpose was work—whether field labor, construction labor, factory labor, house labor, child-rearing labor, farm labor, or domestic labor. Beyond that, a body was a site of either pain or pleasure—illness, exhaustion, dance, sex, et cetera. Alcohol or drugs were either a way to chase pleasure or a way to numb pain. Given the scarcity of resources—in terms of both finances and time—anything else was foolish, meaningless, or an exercise in vanity. Exercise made no sense to people who spent their days engaged in physical labor. Food was to satisfy hunger and to bring pleasure—not primarily for nutrition. Medical care was for injuries and wounds and catastrophic illness—not to maintain or improve health. Life in a consumerist/capitalist society stresses that possessions are paramount and directly correlate to life quality. A vehicle or a home or a television takes precedence over better-quality food or exercise equipment or preventive health care. Add to this the scarcity of time that occurs when working-class/poor people are overwhelmed with multiple jobs, additional travel time due to using public transportation or communal transportation, and family/caregiving responsibilities. In these situations, dedicating the essential resource of time to care for the body often ends up being the last priority.

Along similar lines, in a racist and capitalist society, bodies of color are endlessly devalued. And not just devalued but actively hated. Even as a child, I was called a "dirty Mexican" and a "wetback." I grew up in an emotionally/physically/sexually abusive household. There was no family-based message of value to contest the message of devaluation from mainstream society. Poor. Brown. Female. Devalued and hated on all counts. We internalize these messages in ways that fundamentally shape our lives and our relationships to our bodies. Writing *Blood Sugar Canto,* I kept returning to the thought "I know no one ever told us we were worthy of love." And where else does self-care begin? Where else does valuing the health and strength of our bodies begin? Where else does self-advocacy begin?

We think of voice often when we think of poetry, of writing in general. How do we locate and empower the voices that are authentically ours? How do we find the voice that allows the work, the language, to flow through us? We rarely think about how we find our voices when it comes to our health. How do we tell our loved ones and our coworkers and people on the street that we are diabetic? How do we learn to ask what we need to ask of nurses and doctors and even technicians? What does it take to learn how to stand up for ourselves, our bodies, our lives? To say "This medication is not what I need . . . I need you to listen to me . . . I want to try something else . . . This may be standard protocol but it isn't what I need . . . This is the kind of help I need."

And beyond that, to insist on respect, care, and kindness from health care professionals. To persevere through bureaucratic obstacles, whether with or without health insurance and the funds for co-pays and prescriptions. Where do we find the voice that believes with everything it has that it is necessary to fight for the body?

And so, eleven years into this juggling act, I'm still working on dismantling the underlying beliefs that do not work for me and articulating the ones that I want to inform and shape my life now and in the future. Not fear but love. The priority and purpose of creating art and creating beauty. Value. Self-love. Empowered voice. Gratitude.

There are days where all I do is voice my frustrations, but when I become conscious again, I know that it's gratitude that takes up the greatest part of me. When the juggling reaches overwhelming levels, when I'm tired and in pain, when finances are stretched, when the list of things my brother needs grows too long, what I've learned to do is remember the blessings, the kindnesses of others, the dreams realized and the dreams still nascent.

My brother endured years without medication for his pain, anxiety, or depression. He endured years of extremely limited mobility. He came close to dying and survived a high-risk amputation in 2017. He is still with me now and has medications that make things tolerable. In a way, his wheelchair has given him access to so many things he didn't have for years and years. We came close to losing everything, but community came to our rescue in the absence of family.

We live in an apartment that is cleaner, safer, and more beautiful than anywhere we have lived before. We've both been through doctors and specialists without number and have finally found supportive doctors who work with us. I have bad days and pain days, but this is the strongest and most pain-free I've felt in a decade. As for work, I'm five years away from retiring. The editing/consulting work remains steady. The speaking gigs and class visits are steadily increasing. My fourth book was recently published. I'm working on writing and publishing the next four. In the last decade, we have moved so far from where we were.

Dwelling in the perfect and peaceful moments, minutes, and days gives us the strength to dream the future more deeply. More peace. More health. More strength. More movement. More creation. More art. More beauty. We have come so far that it only makes sense to believe that we can call more beauty and more harmony into our lives.

We live and we persevere, investigating the logic and the belief systems, the assumptions and the truths that undergird every decision, every prioritization of one need over another, every understanding of our days. Living is not a scorecard. Not a matter of how many rules we can follow or how many checklists we can satisfy. Not a matter of exceeding or falling short of other people's expectations or judgments.

My brother and I understand each other. What is healing without freedom? What is life without beauty? Other than caring for ourselves and each other, what else is a more worthy use of our lives than to create?

And so we live, dreaming the perfect moments into being and breathing in those minutes, making ourselves stronger and filling ourselves with their infinity.

• • • •

Author's note: This essay was written in early 2019. My brother, Moisés S. L. Lara, died at home on July 24, 2022, from kidney failure and an infected foot ulcer. A gifted poet, painter, cook, and gardener, he died at age forty. When my time comes, I hope to be buried at his side.

CHAPTER 3

Parenting as a Radical Act of Muxerista Caregiving

Honey and Her Honeybees

ANITA TIJERINA REVILLA

Anita Tijerina Revilla's essay testifies to the barriers between familial caregiver relations, including mental health issues, substance abuse, poverty, and lack of opportunity. In her case, a familial caregiving experience arrangement between the author and her sister's children results in a positive outcome that is achieved as a result of the sacrifices of a living professor aunt.

My cell phone wakes me up. I look at the time. It is 3:00 a.m. It is my sister, again, leaving her sixth message demanding that I answer. She has been texting me all night long. I listen to the messages. She pleads, "Anna, are you okay? Are the kids okay?" "Sister. Please call me back. I can hear the kids screaming. They are crying."

I pick up the next time she calls. "Sister, the kids are fine," I assure her. "They are safe. They are asleep."

She weeps quietly at first, then louder and uncontrollably. Her voice shrieks, "I can hear them, Anna! Don't lie to me!" She quivers and angrily yells into the phone, "I can hear them crying, yelling for help! They need me! I'm going to call the police." She hangs up and calls several times more throughout the night. I do not answer. I fall asleep but never quite feel rested, always feeling something horrible is about to take place.

She doesn't call the police tonight, but she has before. She lives in San Antonio, and we live in Long Beach. She has called the police department in California from her home in Texas to report the children being harmed in our home, even though our kids have assured her that they are safe. I have received these phone calls in the middle of the night hundreds of times. Every time, I fear that someone has been hurt. I wonder, Is someone dead? Did a fight take place? Is my sister hurt, or has my sister hurt my mother? Visions of death and struggle flood my mind. I have lived with a fear of answering the phone at night since I first went away to college and left my family.

I grew up in a home that was filled with love and affirmation, *and* rage and pain. My mom filled us with dreams and assurance that we could succeed, that we could go to college and become anything we dreamed of becoming. She believed in us. I received the message early on that I could use my "school smarts" to pull us out of poverty. I put all my energy into making sure

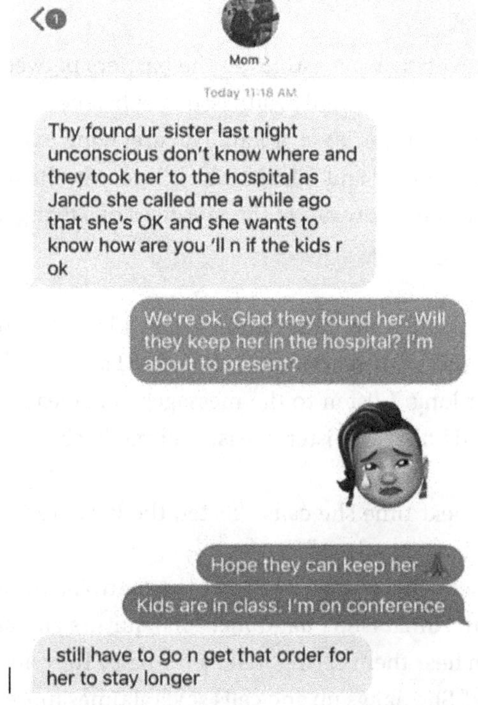

FIGURE 3.1 April 15, 2021, 11:18 a.m., text message from my mother. [My mother's text paraphrased: They found your sister last night unconscious. Don't know where. They took her to the hospital as Jane Doe. She called me a while ago to tell me that she's okay, and she wants to know how you all are, if the kids are okay.]

I could attain this goal. To be certain I could have my chance, I completed every piece of coursework I was ever assigned. I joined and became president of every after-school club that would have me: Future Business Leaders of America *and* Future Homemakers of America, National Honor Society, student council, decathlon, and more.

School has always been easier for me than home. At school, I excelled, and there was little knowledge of the pain we experienced at home. They were separate worlds, and school was my escape. With my mother's support and commitment, I was able to focus on academics. Even though we desperately needed money, she refused to make me work, because school was the most important goal I was expected to pursue. I was indeed afforded the opportunity to attend several elitist universities. Off to Princeton, Columbia, and UCLA I went, far away from the neighborhood I grew up in, including the house whose foundation was caving, the leaky roof, the faulty electric wiring that shut off every time we ran too much electricity at the same time, the yellow walls with holes in the Sheetrock from fights we had over the years, and the tiny, moldy bathroom with an unsteady toilet. When I left, I thought that one day I would buy my mom a house and that she would no longer have to live in this house, but that day has yet to come. My biggest inspiration to get to college was my mom, and activism and the fight for social justice helped me make it through the rest.

Familia

When my father was alive, he was drinking himself to death. My mom says he didn't drink water. All he drank was beer. His preferred beer was Old Milwaukee, but Bud Light was a second favorite. I don't remember a time when he didn't have a beer in his hand. He was a kind father to me. He and I read comics together—Archie and Jughead were our favorite characters in the comics. He was a smart man, an avid reader, and a poet. After college, I was excited when I found an old blue hard-shell suitcase in the shed. It was filled with poems written on old yellow paper that my mother had saved and laminated. After she became a teacher's aide, she laminated everything! He had written poems about being a Chicano, being silenced as a brown man in the United States, and being the son of a woman who did backbreaking laundry work on Lackland Air Force Base. On the other side of the poem, there was a sketch of a brown man with lips zipped shut—silenced. Another poem

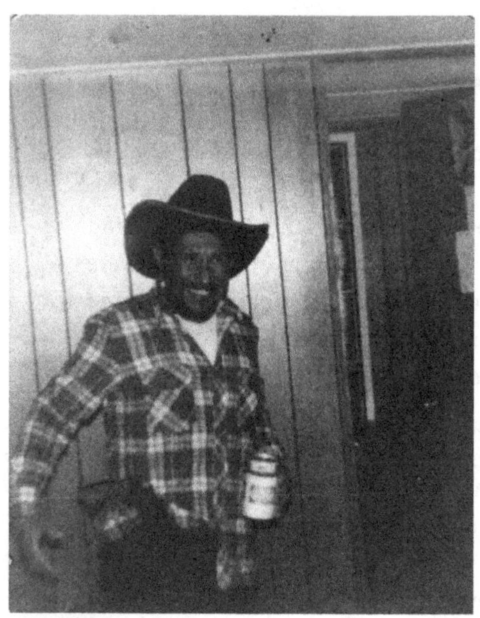

FIGURE 3.2 My father, Luis Arce Revilla, age twenty-nine, circa 1979.

was titled "To My Children . . ." The line I remember the clearest was the line that stated "People will tell you that I was a bad man, the truth is that I was not meant to live in this world."

Those poems opened up a different side of my father to me—one that I never knew or had access to. My father was a sad and angry person, one likely struggling with mental and spiritual illness. He hurt my mom and my brother, so when he died, it was no surprise that my ten-year-old brother had already learned to wield violence against us to demand "respect" in the same way that my father had demanded and taught him. The violence never resulted in us respecting either of them, at least not the violent parts of them. I was grateful my father had died. As early as when I was in third grade, the year he died, I remember thanking God that he was no longer with us and hoping that we could live more freely now that he was gone.[1] My mother was thirty. He was thirty-one years old and had been dying of cirrhosis of the liver. The vehicle he was in was struck by a drunk driver on an April night in 1981. My mom was left to care for three small children on her own, ages three, eight, and ten. She grew stronger before our eyes in my father's absence. She went back to school, earned her GED, became independent, stopped making tortillas on demand, went out dancing to Tejano music with her sisters and friends, didn't let anyone tell her how to live her life, and wore makeup and cowboy boots! Our lives changed, and yet some things stayed the same.

1. bell hooks writes, "Women and children all over the world want men to die so that they can live. This is the most painful truth of male domination, that men wield patriarchal power in ways that are awesomely life-threatening, that women and children cower in fear and various states of powerlessness, believing that the only way out of their suffering, their only hope is for men to die, for the patriarchal father not to come home." See bell hooks, *The Will to Change: Men, Masculinity, and Love* (New York: Atria Books, 2004), 8.

My brother has two children in their early thirties, and my sister gave birth to two children, who are now sixteen and seventeen years old. I did not birth my own children. That was never my plan, but I grew up in a family that depended on all of us being active in the caretaking of the entire family. Primarily, I offered emotional and eventually financial care because I was the nerdy and well-behaved child of the family. When there was a need, I did my best to fulfill it. I did what was asked of me, especially at school. It was my goal in life to take care of my family, and that was the primary reason that I wanted to go to college. I worked hard to go to elitist institutions because of the promise

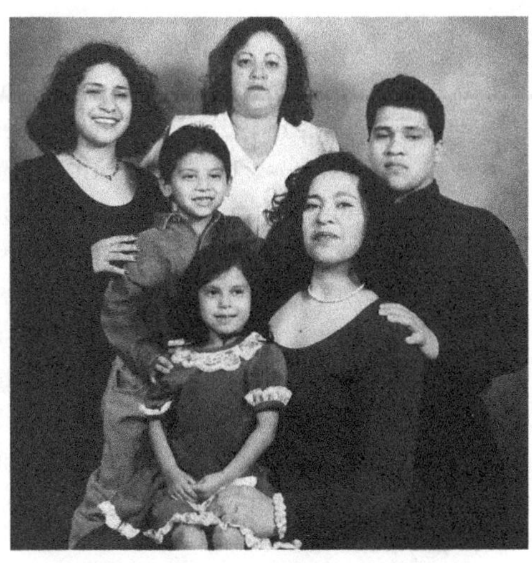

FIGURE 3.3A Family photo with my mom, brother, sister, and brother's children. Top row: my sister, mother, brother. Second row: my nephew and me. Third row: my niece on my lap, circa 1993.

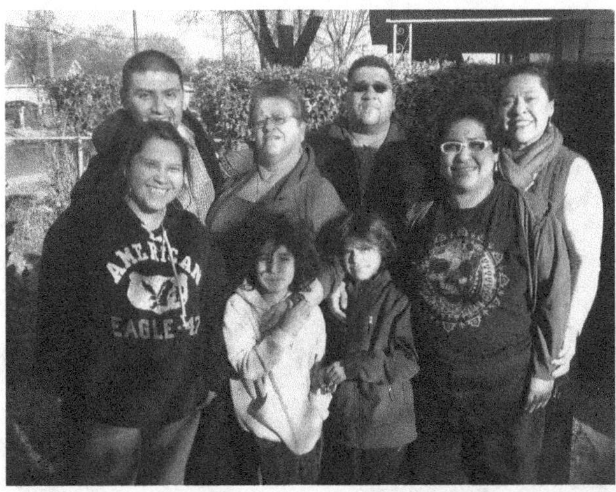

FIGURE 3.3B Photo of my family taken in front of the house we grew up in on the Southside of San Antonio, circa 2012. Top row: my nephew Anthony; my mother, Delia; my brother, Luis; me. Bottom row: my niece Destiny; my nephew Michael; my niece Rae; and my sister, Dee Dee.

that these degrees would allow me to properly care for my family. I wanted to repay my mother for everything she had done for us, and I also wanted to relieve some of the pain she had experienced as a young widow.

I always knew that if something happened to my brother or sister, I would be responsible for helping to care for their children. My mother ended up taking care of my brother's kids, Destiny and Anthony, when their mother died of a drug overdose and a broken heart. I was not ready. I was still in graduate school and could not bring them to live with me. Years later, when my sister, Dee Dee, became too mentally and spiritually ill to care for herself and her children, she asked me to take care of her and the two babies, Rae and Michael, until she was better. I still was not ready to be a parent. I was a brand-new professor on the tenure track, but I could not and would not say no to her.

La Calle Vickers

This picture (figure 3.3b) was taken in front of the house I grew up in on Vickers Avenue in San Antonio, Texas (figure 3.4). We moved into this house after my father died. My mom worked hard to own and care for

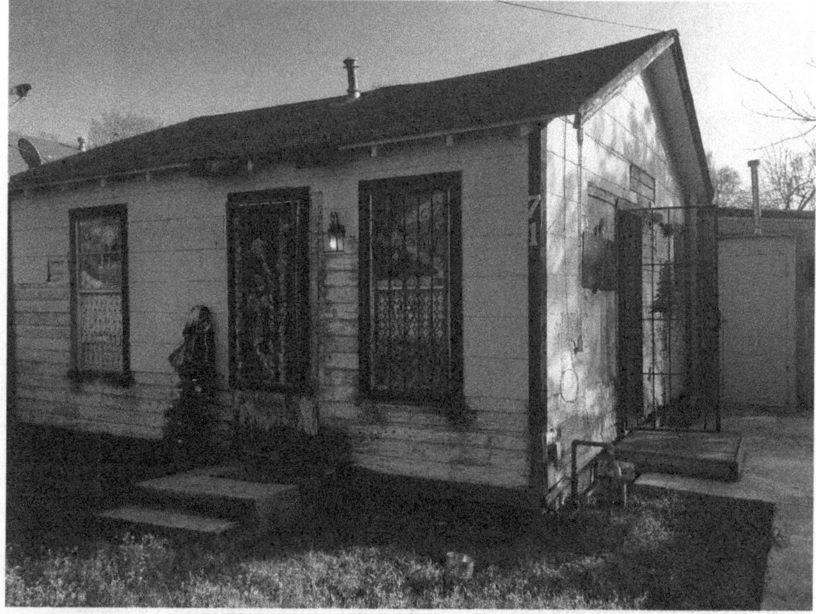

FIGURE 3.4 The house we grew up in. The house my sister still lives in.

that house. My grandfather built the house, and my mom grew up in it as a child. He gave the house to his only son (my uncle Sleepy). When my uncle moved out and into a bigger house, he sold it to my mom because she was recently widowed. He sold it to her for $3,000 in payments. When we moved into the house in 1982, we were on the verge of moving into the Victoria Courts, one of San Antonio's housing projects with the harshest conditions.[2] Instead, we moved into this little house on the Southside of town, near the corner of Southcross Boulevard and Zarzamora. The house was small and falling apart even when we first moved in, but it gave us the stability and home we sorely needed. My mom gave her heart and soul to take care of all three of us. Today, my sister continues to live in that house. It is the place where madness reigns and sadness dominates, and I no longer feel comfortable entering it.

Delia, My Mother

My mother has been my biggest support in life. She is the strongest, funniest, most loyal, most fierce woman I have ever known. Michael, my nephew (and son), says his grandma is the coolest person he knows because she smokes weed, cusses, and loves him like no other. That sums her up well. He also says, "That woman is all about building relationships. She will talk to everyone, and she is always laughing and in a good mood." He becomes thoughtful and says somberly, "She is always hiding her pain." Her journey in life has been long and challenging. Today she is seventy-two years old—still an incredibly spunky and fun mom—one who triggers me regularly. She was kicked out of Catholic elementary school because she spoke out against racist white teachers, nuns from Philadelphia who regularly punished children for speaking Spanish in school and privileged white children over Brown children.

"Shit . . . I told that nun," my mom recalls, "'Why do you even ask us who wants to go to the front office for you? All these little Mexicans always raise their hands, and you *always* pick a white kid.' Her face turned red! She said, 'What are you talking about? Why do you think I am trying to learn Span-

2. See Living New Deal (n.d.) for the history of Victoria Courts. They were demolished in 2000. My first boyfriend grew up in Victoria Courts. He was caught in a crossfire shooting with friends and was convicted of murder of one of the young men who died in the crossfire.

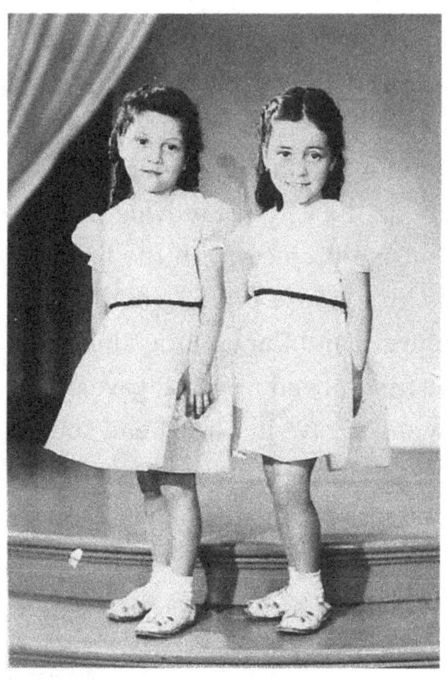

FIGURE 3.5A My *tía* Bea and my mom, ages six and five, circa 1955.

ish?' I said, 'You only want to learn Spanish so you can know what we're saying about you.' She picked up her hand with a ruler in it, and she wanted to hit me with it, but I stopped her! I held her hand and told her, 'If you hit me with that, I'm gonna kick your ass.'" Needless to say, that was the end of Catholic school for my mom.

Her parents, who never had the opportunity to finish school themselves, told my mom, "We don't know why we waste our money sending you to school; you don't even learn nothing." They did not know that she struggled with an undiagnosed learning disability, anxiety, and depression. Eventually, she was pushed out of high school because she married my father. They were not allowed to attend high school as a married couple, and because she was a woman, she was the one who was asked to leave school in the eleventh grade. Because he was a man, he finished high school and received his degree. When he died, she was determined to do all the things my father and her parents did not allow her to do. She enrolled in night school and earned her GED and proceeded to become a licensed security guard.

My mom is a small lady. She is only five feet tall, but she loved the power of walking around with a gun on her belt and telling drunk men they had to leave the bar. And while I am not a gun advocate, I know how much power and autonomy that job gave her. All her life she was told that she could not do certain things because she was a woman. She could not travel, she could not play a musical instrument, she could not join the military, and she could not live an independent, autonomous life. As a woman, she was expected to get married and have children.

When my father died, my mother experienced freedom. She was free from the violence he had inflicted on her, which was rooted in the violence that he had experienced. She was also free from having to answer to anyone else. My mother gave us permission to do anything we wanted, regardless

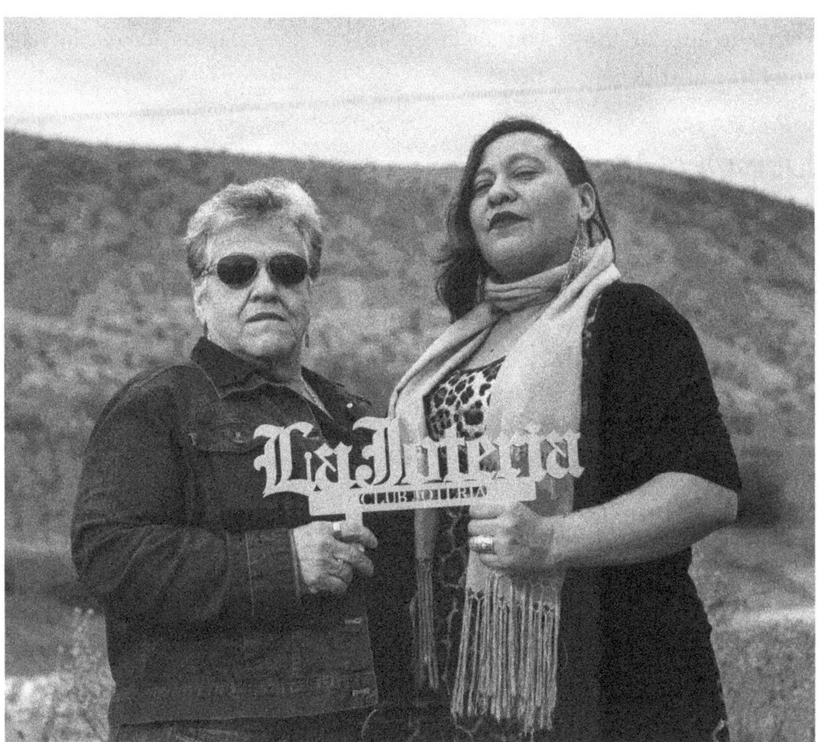

FIGURE 3.5B My mother and me in front of a Las Vegas, Nevada, mountain with an art piece created by Vick Quezada, a lowrider-style *placa* that reads "*La Jotería*," 2017.

of our gender. In fact, her message to us was that because we were women, she was even more determined to give us the freedom to exist as we wished. It was her own special brand of feminism, even though that wasn't what we called it. She never received a formal higher education, but she decided that she would support us to pursue college nonetheless. She sold barbecue plates so I could travel to Washington, D.C., with my class in the seventh grade, and again in twelfth grade so I could buy a flight to New Jersey and start my first year at Princeton. I want to take a moment to remark on her strength and resilience, which you can visually see in her eyes and posture (figure 3.5b).

It took me most of my life to figure out that in spite of all the love and resilience we received and witnessed, there are still deep wounds that have yet to be healed. Those wounds creep up, and they slap us across the face and force us to reconcile them.

Dee Dee, My Sister

> Tell my kids I love them. Tell Mikey I love him. Tell Rae I love her. Tell them I'm sorry for being impolite. I just feel so hurt. I'm so angry. I'm so hurt by society. It's like the time the little girl went down the slide with wet clothes on. And I had to go next. I was so sad, sister. My clothes were all dirty. I just wanted to play. But I couldn't play anymore. Tell my kids I love them. I'm just so scared. Please be careful. Stay away from evil.
>
> —DEE DEE
>
> I will, sister. Pray for peace in your heart.
>
> —ANNA
>
> Even if I have peace in my heart, that doesn't mean that evil stays away from me. How can I keep the evil away? Stay away from me.
>
> —DEE DEE
>
> Pray that you can tell the difference between someone who is evil and trying to hurt you and someone who is not.
>
> —ANNA
>
> I just can't tell anymore. I just want to feel safe. Tell my kids I love them. I love you, sister.
>
> —DEE DEE
>
> I love you, sister.
>
> —ANNA
>
> [CONVERSATION BETWEEN MY SISTER AND ME, NOVEMBER 5, 2020, 7:31 A.M.]

My sister, who is four years younger than me, was diagnosed with bipolar and schizoaffective disorder fourteen years ago, in 2008. She had a deep mental health breakdown. Some might say that she "went mad." Quite literally, all the sadness she had experienced in her life—the loss of our father; poverty; physical and sexual abuse; racism; sexism; classism; abusive friends, family, and partners; and finally the loss of her child drove her to madness. She was pregnant with her first child and lost her baby at six months. The baby had not finished forming when she gave birth to her. The doctor said that the baby was falling apart in his hands as he delivered her. All the hurt and betrayal she had ever experienced, all the loss, could no longer be contained,

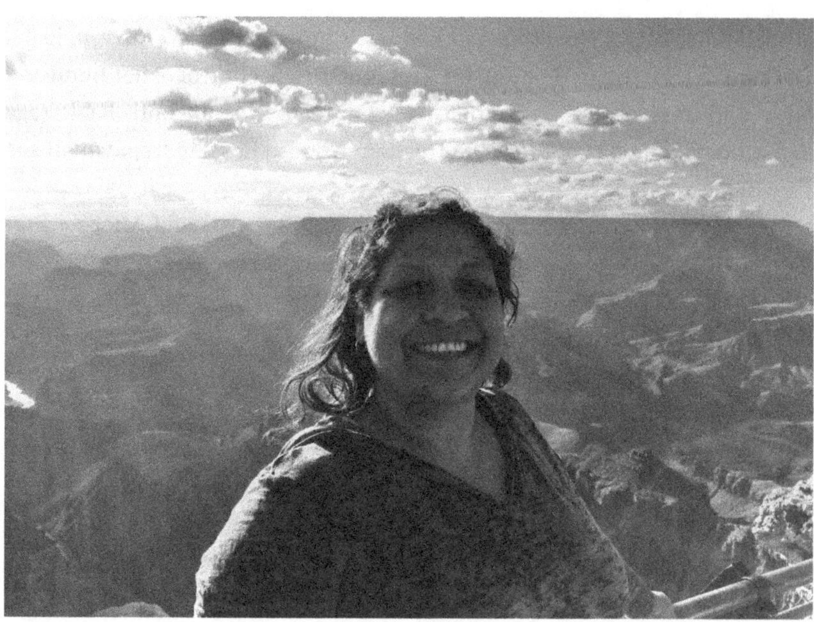

FIGURE 3.6A My sister standing in front of the Grand Canyon, 2014.

and it was released in a complete state of madness and rage. The filter that she'd had for the first thirty years of her life was slowly being ripped off, and she could no longer contain it. She could no longer hold it together, as if she were saying "Because of all of the hurt I have experienced, I cannot go one step further without telling you how angry I am at the world, at myself, and at the people around me." I saw her begin to cycle into manic episodes of extreme happiness and joy and extreme hurt and anger.

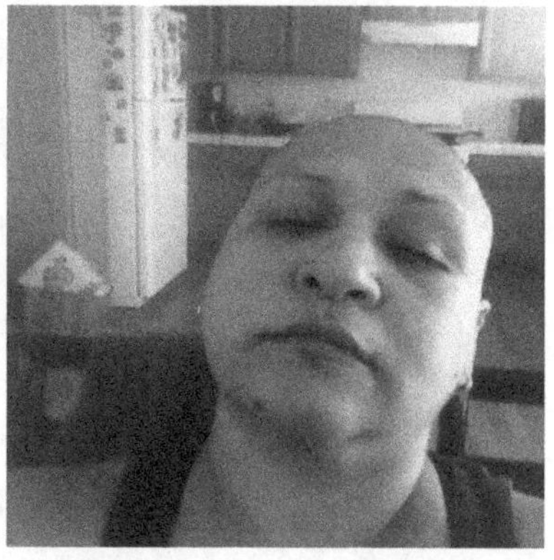

FIGURE 3.6B My sister in my dining room after unexpectedly deciding to shave her head, 2014.

These photos exhibit some of what Dee Dee was experiencing internally (figures 3.6a and 3.6b). She is an extremely intelligent and strong woman. She was studying history and Chicana/o studies, was pursuing a career as a librarian, was on the dean's list at the University of Houston, and had just transferred to UT Austin, just a few credits short of graduation. But this illness took control of her mind and body, and the freedom to live her life is limited by the uncontrollable rage and sadness. She has not had the freedom to raise her children, which she very much wanted.

After losing her first baby, she gave birth to Rae Ana and Michael (figure 3.7). Her husband, Jason, was selling marijuana to keep them afloat, while smoking every day, all day—self-medicating. He is a survivor of childhood physical and emotional abuse. He was diagnosed with schizophrenia at the age of twelve, around the same age that his brother was murdered and took his last breath in his arms. When Rae was two years old and Michael was one, Dee Dee and her husband could no longer sustain their relationship. Jason left, and my sister started hustling to take care of herself and the kids. She took over Jason's hustle, and slowly, her world began to spin and eventually crumble. When Rae was three and Jason had left already, she was listening to an Alicia Keys song, a song that Rae and Dee Dee both loved. Alicia Keys belted out these lines:

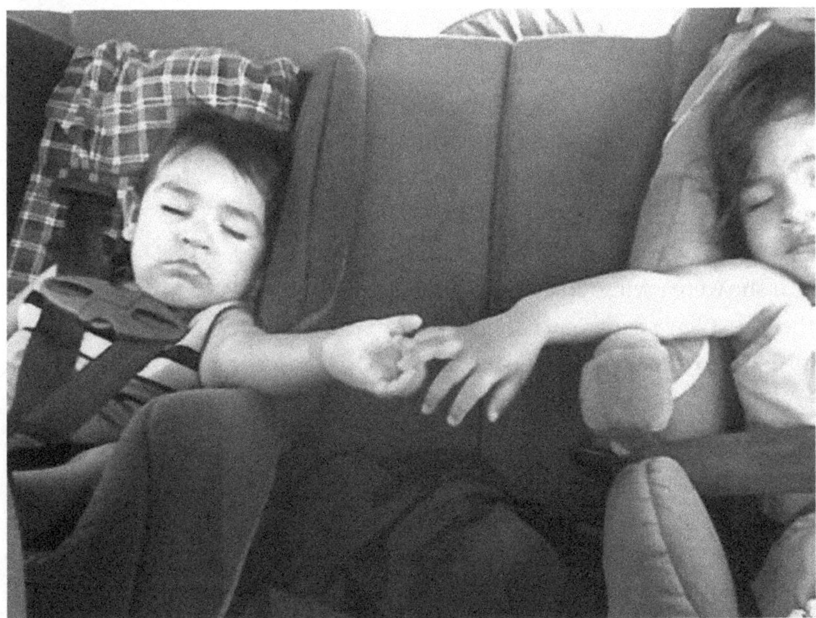

FIGURE 3.7 Michael and Rae in the back seat of the car when they still lived in Texas, circa 2007.

No one, no one, no one
Can get in the way of what I'm feeling
No one, no one, no one
Can get in the way of what I feel for you, you, you . . .

As they listened, Rae said to her mom, "Dad broke my heart, Mom." It was a heartbreak my sister could resonate with deeply, but her pain was caused not only by Jason but by many other hardships she had experienced in her lifetime. My sister was renting the house behind my mom's house. The kids were still in diapers. They had a makeshift ladder that the babies used to climb the fence to visit their grandma. Rae was a master climber at the time. Drug users and dealers came in and out of their house, and my sister was working hard to take care of herself, the babies, my mom, and even my older niece.

My sister's voice became more and more distant. She called me less, and when she did, she talked nonstop, a million words a minute, it seemed like. She talked about Jesus, her Christian beliefs, and the harm that people were trying to do to her. There was a man she loved in the neighborhood. He was her boyfriend, and he kept hurting and mistreating her. One day, my mother called me and told me that my sister had thrown away every one of her possessions. She had put them all out on the curb—televisions, furniture, clothes, jewelry, everything. She said that she had to get rid of them because they had been purchased with dirty money. She told us that God was coming for her and that she was ready. She regularly spoke to religious and spiritual figures who either judged her or gave her advice. The delusions had begun. Not knowing what to do, my mother called the police to take her to the hospital. My sister was furious. My mom found her in the closet of her house, waiting for God to come for her.

The next incident was more severe. She was looking for her boyfriend at his house down the street. She was screaming at him and his family. She told me that they had stolen money from her or owed her money they had borrowed. Fearful of her, I assume, they called the police on her. When they arrived, she was crossing the street, Zarzamora, to go to the corner store. The police questioned her in her state of madness. I was told that she screamed at them to be left alone, and because police authorities have no mental health training, and especially didn't in 2008, they beat her with their clubs and threw her in jail.

I flew home to try to help. I went to the county jail, and for over a week, they refused to let me see her. I assumed it was because her bruises were fresh and gruesome. I tried to explain to them that she was mentally ill but to no avail. I hired a lawyer, who helped me get the charges dropped, and they transferred her to a state hospital. It was the first time she was getting officially hospitalized for her mental illness. It would be the first time she received medication beyond antidepressants. I flew back to Las Vegas to go back to work and waited. The babies were three and four years old. My sister was thirty-one years old. (She just turned forty-five.) When she came out of the hospital, she called me and said, "I'm gonna need your help, sister. I need you to take care of me and the babies." She flew to Vegas with the kids. After a couple of months, she went back to San Antonio and left me alone with the babies.

I did not want to do it. I did not want to be a parent. I had worked really hard to not become a teen parent or single parent, as many young women in my community were expected to become, and had instead focused on school and my career.[3] I had spent all my life taking care of my family—my sister, my brother's kids, and my mom. I am the only one who is financially stable and has the ability to take care of multiple family units. That I was prepared for, but I was not prepared for what it takes to become a full-time parent to two toddlers, and so began my journey of coming to terms with becoming a *tía-mamá*, or, as the kids like to call me, Honey.[4] My entire life changed. I had been a young, untenured professor who woke up at noon and went to bed at 3:00 or 4:00 a.m. My road to healing had not yet begun. I was completely focused on work, activism, and community. I loved my family and provided economically and emotionally to the best of my ability, but this would be very different. Caregiving as a muxerista parent would be the revolutionary journey I could never have imagined.

---

3. I want to make clear that I am not judging teen or single parents. As a person raised by a single mom and who is friends with several teen moms, I know their determination, resilience, and strength. I also am aware of their incredible struggles.

4. When I was in middle school, my cousin and his girlfriend had a baby named Samantha. They were our neighbors and teen parents. I spent a lot of time helping to take care of Sammy Jo. I used to call her my little honey, so when she first learned to talk, she called me *onnie*, or "honey." The nickname stuck, and every family baby who was born after her called me Honey as well. The kids have always called me Honey, but it was a perfect term, given my status as both tía and mom to them. Since we have always been clear that my sister is their birth mom and I am their tía and their primary parent, *Honey* is a perfect compromise—it signifies that I am more than Tía but not necessarily Mother. It honors our bond and intimate connection as well as their mom's continued presence and role in their lives.

Passenger Information			
Passenger Name	Account Number	Ticket#	Expiration[1]
MCMURREN/MICHAEL ANTHONY	- None Entered -	526-8511338349-0	08/24/09

[1] All travel involving funds from this Confirmation Number must be completed by the expiration date.

Itinerary		
Date	Flight	Routing Details
Sat Oct 18	1981	Depart SAN ANTONIO TX (SAT) at 2:15 PM Arrive in LAS VEGAS NV (LAS) at 3:10 PM

Passenger Information			
Passenger Name	Account Number	Ticket#	Expiration[1]
MCMURREN/RAE ANA	- None Entered -	526-8511337889-2	10/16/09

[1] All travel involving funds from this Confirmation Number must be completed by the expiration date.

Itinerary		
Date	Flight	Routing Details
Sat Oct 18	1981	Depart SAN ANTONIO TX (SAT) at 2:15 PM Arrive in LAS VEGAS NV (LAS) at 3:10 PM

FIGURE 3.8 Southwest flight receipts for Rae and Michael's flight to Las Vegas, October 18, 2008.

Codependent Parenting No More[5]

I have to admit that while my mother is an amazing parent and fierce woman, she is also a codependent parent. Most of us have seen this kind of parenting, have lived it, or are living in it currently. It can look like trying to control other people's behavior in an attempt to help them while neglecting yourself. It can look like giving people unwanted advice and trying to change other people instead of yourself. It can look like trying to take care of everyone except yourself, at your expense.

There are many characteristics of codependent behavior, but it was not until a friend of mine was diagnosed with codependence that I learned about it. I was jokingly complaining that another friend, who was in the hospital, did not let me stay at her house when I needed a place to stay, and I joked that if it were me, I would have offered my keys and told my friend to stay at my house even while I was in the hospital. My friend answered, "Of course you would because you are codependent!" She opened up the book she was reading, and as I read through the characteristics of codependence, I was

5. See Beattie 1987.

horrified to see myself in them, and at the same time, I realized that I was often praised for many of the characteristics that were listed.

Typically, a codependent person is one who is overreliant on the value placed on them by a partner, usually a partner who is ill or addicted. The codependent person's value is determined by their ability to "save" or help their partner. I have experienced this in a romantic relationship, *and* I have also seen signs of codependency in my friendships, activism, and familial and work relationships. Because my family struggles so much with mental illness, as well as racism, poverty, patriarchy, and other forms of structural abuse, I have often prioritized their needs above my own, and I have felt the need to "save" them, even when they did not ask to be saved. I have questioned my value and felt guilty when I have not been able to help them, even if I myself am struggling and unable to get help for myself.

I witnessed codependent partnering and parenting from most of the women in my life—my mom, grandmother, aunts, and cousins. I witnessed my mom in a codependent relationship with her parents. Even though her mother and father often criticized her and rejected her sense of self and freedom, they loved her and depended on her to help care for them, especially as they aged and became ill. My mother was my grandmother's caretaker until the latter's recent death. Both my sister and brother are emotionally abusive to my mother at times (which is complicated because both of them experienced abuse growing up), and my mother enables their behavior and is loyal to serving their needs. Her value as a mom is determined by how much she does for them. When I have told my mother that I do not want to follow these practices, she has felt betrayed and unloved. I fall out of favor when I voice these feelings. She has fully internalized the codependent parenting model. It is affirmed by all, even outside our family, in pop culture and the mainstream. A good mother is self-sacrificing. Her value is embedded in the ways that she serves her family, so my mom was mostly confused by my rejection of codependent parenting.

My mother sacrificed herself to ensure that we were cared for. She never remarried. In fact, she sabotaged relationships with potential partners so that she could focus on our needs. Often she would boast that she told men to go to hell: "I told him, 'My kids come first!'" As a result, she entered old age with much loneliness. She lost sight of her desires and need for pleasure so that she could give us all her attention and the limited resources she had. Many people say that the best kind of mother is a self-sacrificing mother, the kind who will not focus on her own needs so that she can meet her children's needs. However, there is a thin line between the ideal all-loving, self-sacrificing mother and the patriarchal expectation that a woman/mother should not value herself or her needs but should instead focus on her husband's/partner's and children's needs. This kind of woman should not be an independent, autonomous person. She should have no space for fun or love that is not connected to her children or partner.

For instance, my mom would not even go out to eat at a fast-food restaurant without us because she felt so much guilt. To this day, she continues these practices even though we are all grown, living our own lives and enjoying simple pleasures without her. Today, she struggles to figure out how to live her own life independently of her children and grandchildren. Even for fun or a meal, she cannot bring herself to partake without considering everyone else's desires and needs. She is having a hard time figuring out what might bring joy to her life, which is increasingly important because her mother just passed away and my sister's illness worsens daily. Instead, she often stays in a place of sadness and isolates herself when she is not providing care for others. She no longer dances or goes out to listen to music. It makes her too sad because she cannot dance without being in physical pain, but she also is always too busy taking care of others.

I realize now that my mother parented us through lenses of wounding and codependence. She did not have a model for healing and had no idea that she could prioritize her own physical and spiritual health while parenting us. As I became a parent, I sought a different model of parenting. I worked to identify the patriarchal patterns and expectations of women, mothers, and parents and tried to do the opposite. My mother had already laid some of the groundwork for me at a young age. With the help of a former partner and my muxerista and *jotería* community, I found and co-created a model for parenting that was rooted in self and collective healing. It is very much connected to the social justice vision that I have outlined in my academic work on muxerista and jotería community.[6] Muxerista and jotería parenting is Chicanx/Latinx feminist, queer, radical caretaking rooted in loving and healing the self and the collective. Moreover, muxerista and jotería caretaking practices harm reduction and antiviolence in and outside the home and

6. See the tenets of muxerista pedagogy and jotería identity and consciousness and apply to parenting and family building.

seeks an end to patriarchy, racism, homophobia, transphobia, ableism, and codependence.

Parenting Is a Radical Act of Muxerista Caregiving

Today, I am still working to do my best to raise young human beings who are deeply connected to a foundation of love, healing, authenticity, and humanization. I am no longer resisting being a parent. I am honored to have had the opportunity to raise these fierce beings and to be their Honey, tía, and parent. I have fully consented and embraced my role as their parent and caregiver in partnership with my sister, my mom, and my community. Rae and Michael do not want me to replace their mom. They want me to help their mom raise them because she is sick, heartbroken, and spirit murdered. I do my best to help her while keeping in mind that I also need to balance her care with my own care. I pay for her housing costs. I try to keep her as safe as possible, given her life filled with madness and addiction, and most important, I am the primary caretaker of *our* children. I have never told her or had the desire to tell her that Rae and Michael are my children and not hers—to do so would be to shatter the last bit of hope and love left in her heart. I am clear with the teens that their mother, my sister, will always be their mother. She loves them deeply and has made the biggest sacrifice a mother can make when she is too ill to care for her children: to choose a safer caretaker for them than herself. She entrusted them to me because she knew they would be safe with me. They are *our* children. I am both tía and legal mom. I adopted them last year to ensure that our legal rights were secure and that no one could take them from me and my muxerista-jotería community if something were to happen to me.

Rae just turned eighteen years old. She is graduating from high school, wants a VW Bug, and is trying to get her license. She loves her new puppy, Gio—she is a huge animal lover. She is testing her limits and trying out being an adult. She is deciding between Cal State Fullerton or Long Beach for college. Michael will turn seventeen this month. He loves metal music, is currently curious about Hinduism, and wants to become an entrepreneur. He wants to own a music store one day and design guitars. He is very close to Rae. I am not sure what he will do when she moves away for college. Both were hit hard by the pandemic and lost interest in school, but they are working to bring up all their grades. Luckily, this year, their friends are reconnecting with them. Both hesitate to identify as feminists, but they have a sophisticated feminist critique and social justice foundation that guides them to be better people, and they are far more healed than myself growing up.

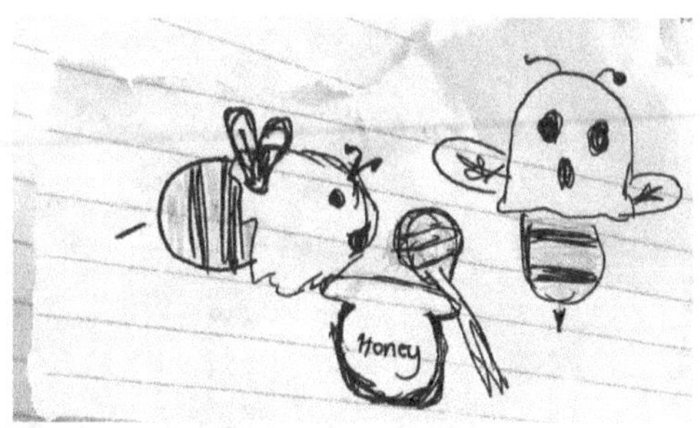

FIGURE 3.9A A drawing by Rae that represents me and her and Michael, 2021.

My mom is finally acknowledging that she is also codependent, after several years of denying it. She is still taking care of my sister, my brother, and her grandkids in Texas, often at her own expense, but once in a while she will take a day off and let me know she is tired and needs to "stop being a codependent." She laughs and starts all over again the next day.

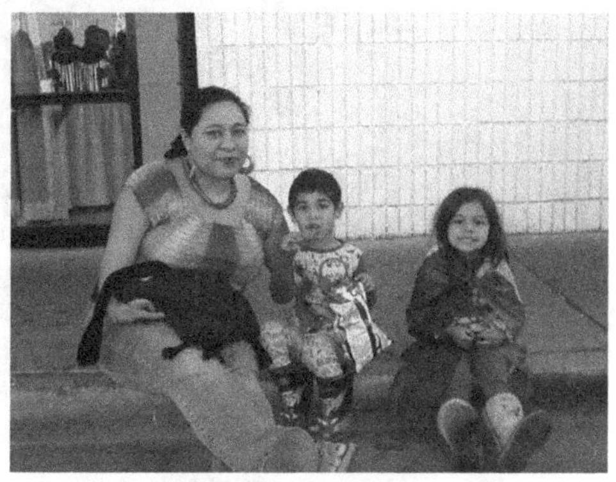

FIGURE 3.9B The kids and me at our first protest in defense of gay marriage / queer community, 2008.

Sadly, this is not a story that culminates in a happy ending. There is no resolution in this story. I often wake up sad and go to sleep sad with my sister on my mind, wishing for a different reality for her. Her illness is at its worst. The pandemic hit her the hardest in our family. She has not received proper health care. Her psychiatrist broke up with her at the beginning of the pandemic because she screamed at him, which is a symptom of her illness, so she has not been on the medications for her diagnosis for almost three years. This has led to increased delusions, paranoia, and aggressive behavior that resulted in an arrest. We are awaiting her court day, hoping she is not further criminalized for her illness. I feel like I am watching her slowly die, maybe even slowly kill herself by self-medicating with unauthorized drugs. I don't know what else to do except to keep providing her love, food, housing, medical care if she will accept it, and a deepening commitment to the caretaking of our children. I miss my little sister. I miss her laughter. I miss her joy, and I am grateful to her for teaching me so much. She has taught me how to love deeper and be

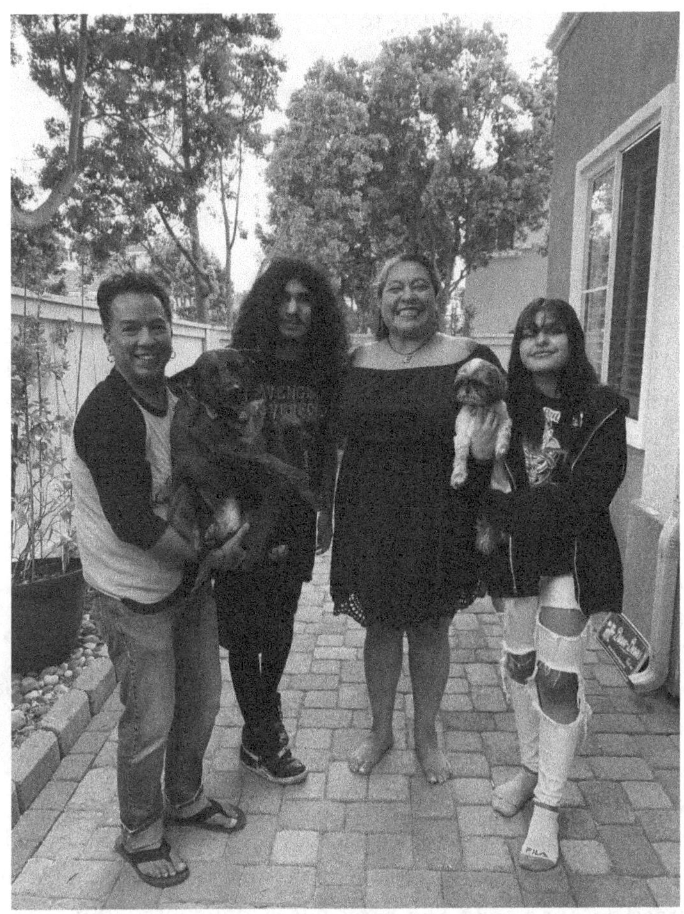

FIGURE 3.9C Veronica (my partner), Michael, me, Rae, and our dogs, Mona and Mabel, visiting family in San Diego, 2020.

vigilant about my healing and our family's healing. Ultimately, she is responsible for me learning how to become a radical muxerista caretaker.

References

Beattie, Melody. 1987. *Codependent No More: How to Stop Controlling Others and Start Caring for Yourself.* New York: Harper and Row.

Living New Deal. n.d. "Victoria Courts—San Antonio TX." Accessed May 15, 2021. https://livingnewdeal.org/projects/victoria-courts-san-antonio-tx/.

CHAPTER 4

Tele-caregiving

A Lifetime of Regenerative Pláticas

ANGIE CHABRAM

Angie Chabram's retrospective introduces important situational and familial practices of caregiving rendered by different generations of Latinas/Chicanas within the Americas daily. While highlighting a communicative role of technology (in this case tele-caregiving), she does not reduce caregiving to this medium. Instead, she focuses on the messages (or the *pláticas*) that are made possible through a lifetime of nourishing female-centered exchanges that are generated over time and place. Her essay also alerts its readers to the need to attend to the dynamic aspect of caregiving and its multiple forms. As her story demonstrates, it is necessary to adapt to situational contexts. In her case she must change to an in-person mode and contend with the limits on speech. She must be not only flexible but also creative, imagining how a culturally relevant communication board or a visual practice can help produce exchanges even when much-needed technologies do not. She foresees future interdisciplinary collaborations where artists, speech therapists, and narratives of health can join forces to produce these much-needed mediums that work together to break the silence.

In their recent article entitled "Who Is Taking Care of the Caregiver?," Amy Sullivan Burleson and Deborah Miller repeat the much-cited proviso "Caregivers must learn to take care of themselves physically and emotionally" (2015, 7). While I agree, I wonder why society doesn't embrace more of the burden of care and lessen individual burnout. I am troubled by state-of-the-art descriptions of caregiving that erase multidisciplinary models already in existence in communities of color, which remain unrecognized. These models offer diverse ways in which giving and receiving care are in place and often incorporate networks of *promotores/as* (a slew of community members who administer health). What is most bothersome to me, however, are the normative binaries of caregiving that presuppose that those who administer care are not the ones who also receive care from those they care for. These binaries ignore the fact that caregiving is a fluid, dynamic intersectional practice, often shared and co-constructed by different social subjects who are susceptible to burnout as well as mutual support and renewal.

Armed with these critical insights, I turned to the topic of this essay and sought relevant sources that could help me understand the unique form of caregiving I had experienced over a lifetime in conjunction with my beloved mother (Angie G. Chabram, 1926–2018). Ironically, instead of finding instances of regenerative forms of interpersonal communication between family members or friends within different locations, I found increasing technological and privatized forms of care, which included surveillance systems that monitored the movements of the recipients of care, tracking lone individuals and alerting them when the alarm (upon a fall, for instance) sounded. In this model of caregiving, it seemed that every effort was made to create a substitute for a model of care based on physical human presence and to opt for a clinical model of caregiving with the outsourcing of care to a number of centers. In these centers family members and paid caregivers with no relationship to the care recipient other than that of employee/employer are predominant. As recent descriptions of these care modalities explain,

> In a tele-caregiving situation, strategically placed video cameras and sensors enable a tele-caregiver to keep tabs on an elder without physically being in their house. Computers and the Internet are also used to enable a family member of the elder or a tele-caregiver to directly communicate with an elder over video chat. (Botek, n.d.)

The problem with this description is that tele-caregiving is more than keeping tabs on an elder while not being in the house with them. Not enough is said about the quality of the communication or the history that has evolved over time, space, and telephone (for instance) that enables the potential afforded by overlapping forms of care in community. In my case, what I was in search of was not surveillance, not a game of hide-and-seek but a description of the *plática,* which I found centered in familial activities, as did Guajardo and Guajardo (2013, 160–61):

> We talk daily, pláticamos on the phone. Plática is a chief modality. . . . [It] is at the root of how we work and live our lives . . . We learned plática—an expressive cultural form shaped by listening, inquiry, storymaking that is akin to nuanced multi-dimensional conversations—from our parents . . . Pláticas were key to allow relationship to flourish, and trust to build within relationships.

I did not want to stress a decontextualized technology (in this case the phone; it was a tool for generating plática).

The source that would lead me to writing my alternative care narrative was none other than Sergio Troncoso's story "La Abuela" (1999). In that El Paso–based story, an elder border grandmother tele-caregives Arturo, who is in the throes of social alienation at Harvard University and needs her for continued academic and spiritual survival. Her telephone calls are pláticas that allow him to appreciate the worth in her life and to find self-respect in a competitive academic environment. Her care involves listening, questioning, advising, providing a voice, counterpoint, and a memory, and actually doing things such as praying on his behalf or initiating a community prayer circle. Here, as in celebrated texts such as Henri Nouwen's *A Spirituality of Caregiving* (2011), reciprocity is important. In the case of "La Abuela," the grandson's phone calls are check-in calls, which his grandparents are eager to receive. As elders who live alone and on government assistance, these calls provide a valuable connection to the outside world and family. In this way grandparents and son form a close-knit circle of support, notwithstanding the geographical and professional distance between them.

Sergio Troncoso's story had a big impact on me because it allowed me to see that my mother and I would develop a similar circle of tele-caring upon my departure for college, graduate school, and professorship. We made *familia* from scratch, defying the distances between us as well as limiting the incursion of the academy into our lives. These mutually sustaining phone calls meant everything to me as I moved from an undergraduate to a professor in the University of California system. We also reveled in our long pláticas about health, family issues, politics, aging, men, and whatever we fancied, including *chisme* (gossip). Truth be told, my mother and I could not get enough. Our phone calls were not only very consistent but were also multiple and always filled with meaningful conversation and exchange. We called each other as a way of grounding ourselves in our relationship, native community, and family and as a way of finding mutual support when health, educational, and societal dynamics were simply not there to sustain us. Like those of the character in Troncoso's story, our phone calls allowed for certain forms of healing and wellness and witnessing to happen that were not available to us in society or in the educational institution of which I formed a part. They allowed us to build a bridge between the community and the academy and to maintain a loving relationship that was in many ways unique. After all, we weren't just any mother and daughter.

We were both named Angie, and we tele-caregave each other for around fifty years, until my mother passed away. We needed mutual support because in many ways our lives had been nontraditional. She was a single parent of four children, and I was a daughter without children. A big part of our connection was providing the kind of support for our unique situations that made us both feel that we were living perfectly normal lives. (This in a Latina/o context that prizes a different form of familism.) As a budding feminist, I reveled in how she came to narrate her unique path of womanhood with pride and gusto and how she would count her successes in human terms, which included how she was able to survive and even thrive with her four children in tow even when her husband had literally abandoned the family. This was no small feat. She began her journey into independence in the fifties, and she not only entered the workforce as a factory worker but made sure her kids got an education too. In my case, oh, she pushed me hard and she heeded my brother's advice, which was that I should do a BA, an MA, and a PhD. She had high hopes for me, and I would not let her down. I marched forward with a lion in my heart. In my long periods of being single, she never pressured me to get married, never pressured me to have children. She did this even though she herself did not have a role model for educating a daughter like this. She pushed me out of the cage and said, "Fly, I got you."

It worked. If I was the first woman in my Chicana/o family to get a doctorate, I was one of the few Chicana professors at UC Davis, and she was one of the first Chicana mothers to guide her daughter along this amazing path, supporting me along with prayers and encouragement and the idea that there was no turning back for either of us, no matter how tough it got.

Failure was not an option; neither was depending on gender myths that had women looking elsewhere for economic support and the guarantee of lifetime companionship. I could not ignore her example or her stories. Hadn't she supported her kids on her own? Didn't she walk to the store with four kids in tow, each with a bag so we could have dinner? Didn't she make us enchiladas, *arroz con frijoles*, chorizo, and *papitas fritas*? Didn't she manage to purchase a house on her paltry salary? Send her kids to Catholic school? Defy the odds over and over again and talk back to stereotypes of the fifties and sixties about would happen to the children and wives of divorce? Didn't all her children obtain leadership positions? Hadn't she told other women who were single parents that they could make it too?

They say the light shines through the wound, and this was true for her, and it was true for both of us. Our light shone bright through our wounds, and we developed the most amazing form of pláticas that enabled her to contend with the loss of a husband and me to contend with the loss of a father. For us we were both enough, *punto*. Eventually the deep wound moved to the rearview mirror, and the light grew brighter and brighter. We thrived for decades. But this did not take away my sense of injustice; I was angry because of all that had been sacrificed and all that I believed life still owed her. She was and always will be my shero. No, another description is in order: She is my Virgen de Guadalupe. She is a new reiteration of the Guadalupe elders that Yolanda López painted in her famous series.

Recently another sense of injustice emerged in the months prior to the passing of my beloved mother at age ninety-two. Not long after this event, I went to clear my answering machine, and I heard my mom trying to say "Hi, Angie." My heart broke. What an injustice; this powerful conversationalist's voice was waning. A month had gone by since her passing, and I felt the terrible loss of my lifelong best friend and ally. My beautiful sister had put her on the phone, and I knew the effort it took to say "Hi, Angie." My heart was heavy. She had really struggled with her speech for a while. This had killed me. The voice was our primary means of communication, and it had been fading.

In desperation I had turned to the internet, searching for a solution and someone or something to help me out. I'd finally settled on a communication chart that had pictures of everyday life events, not phrases from conversations. I was at a point where I could take medical leave for my mom, and I replaced the phone calls with in-person visits. The caregiving had radically changed. I had to train myself to administer care and learn how to listen to decipher her messages through a medley of sounds and to supplement language with movements. I drew on all the strength of my passion and training as a language teacher. I went to the dollar store, and I found some cards. I wrote words on them, and my mom humored me with repetitions. Amid it all she almost always said "I love you," which was all I wanted to hear. Sometimes she'd just break into the most fluent sentences ever. Boy, did I appreciate those surprises.

In retrospect I realize that I really needed to develop more communication skills, especially if I wanted to be of service to Latinas like Mom who struggled with speech. Something had to change. Or would we just accept the silence even when we knew that many aging Latinas had a monumental fear of becoming silent? Things had to change, but I did not know where to start. To begin with, I could imagine my own bilingual communication board, filled with real-life pictures of women like my mom doing things that they always loved to do. I could image them in their favorite clothes, eating Mexican food (tortillas, pan dulce), embracing their children, sitting in the middle of the living room, lying in color-filled rooms with pictures of their ancestors, or praying or listening to music.

I would also have to incorporate the image of them holding someone's hand or being held in return, sitting together with loved ones or beloved animals at a table. Outside of this communication-board reconfiguration, I could imagine myself teaching a course on narrative health and inviting art students to help devise alternative communication boards and maybe inviting the technologically savvy ones to help me record voices for posterity. Maybe having the twenty-four-seven caregiver who communicates with elders who struggle with speech provide feedback to us all would be helpful. After all, from what I witnessed, it is the full-time caregivers who must master new tools of communication and presence on a daily basis. These are the ones we need to hear from as we create venues for learning and speaking and reimagining liberatory dialogues spoken in embodied languages we cannot yet fully imagine.

As I conclude this essay, I realize how privileged I was because my pláticas with my mother not only provided the basis for mutual care but also provided me with a sense of direction in my scholarship. It was because of her that I studied Spanish, because of her that I got into Chicana/o studies, because of her that I delved into Chicana working-class feminism, because of her that I helped compose narratives of health and healing. And now because of her I continue my forays into caregiving, speech therapy, and El Paso literature. Even though she is now in the spirit world, I continue to seek her direction and to fuel my notions of care with her lessons and pláticas about what is truly needed and appreciated.

When I think about the challenges that lie ahead for me, I just think of her last message to me on the phone, where she mustered up all the strength she had, spoke through the difficulties, and said "Hi, Angie." Now I listen for that greeting. Without telephone and speaking board, my body is now the vessel that facilitates her remembrance and the lifelong lessons that guide me as I reimagine my story in relation to the other meaningful intersectional caregiving contexts that tell the bulk of a caregiving story of my mom. These include primary family caregivers present around my mom's place of habitation who were consistently there throughout the years, readily available to clothe, feed, and transport Mom; to have in-person visits with her and friends, organize the family celebrations, help her heal, advocate for her in presence of doctors, and create multiple and stories and reflections.

When I look at these labor-intensive contexts, I realize that my tele-caregiving experiences were a part of a bigger picture that was necessary for care to happen. I realize that I had certain work privileges that afforded a distance from many of the urgent demands of the task. Also, my tele-caregiving context was preceded by a mother and grandmother who had a history of caregiving one another by phone from El Paso to La Puente. In her life, Mom had a history of professional work that included care. As I state elsewhere (Chabram 2006), she quit school to support her father when he broke his spine, worked at the army base at Fort Bliss during World War II, and comforted the wounded. At home she developed a collaborative practice of caregiving within the family between herself and her children, which continues to this day, and gave birth to the regenerative pláticas that sustain us in her absence.

It is not surprising that my three decades of work in Chicana/o studies also involved care collaborations with students, family, and staff; that my siblings and I have continued to search for new methods of connection and outreach; that our pláticas have taken us to new and exciting paths. From my reflections I realize that the forms of caregiving I learned from my mother are akin to what Richards (2009) refers to as "caresharing"; it is practiced in relation to other people and their contributions. In addition, even in group settings, the administration of care is always different: it assumes its form in relation to what is needed and can be given and who the subjects of care are. That is why despite the collaborations that kept us afloat when we became a single-parent family, each one of use cared for one another and the whole differently. That is why the similarities and differences matter.

References

Botek, Anne-Marie. n.d. "Telecaregiving: Be There for an Elder Without Physically Being There." AgingCare. Accessed November 30, 2023. https://www.agingcare.com/articles/tele-caregiving-be-there-for-an-elder-without-physically-being-there-146398.htm.

Chabram, Angie. 2006. "Angie González Chabram." In *Latinas in the United States: A Historical Encyclopedia*, edited by Vicki L. Ruiz and Virginia Sánchez Korrol. Bloomington: Indiana University Press.

Guajardo, Francisco, and Miguel Guajardo. 2013. "The Power of the Plática." *Reflection* 13, no. 1 (Fall): 159–64.

Nouven, Henri J. M., and John S. Mogabgab. 2011. *A Spirituality of Caregiving*. Nashville: Upper Room.

Richards, Marty. 2009. *Caresharing: A Reciprocal Approach to Caregiving and Care Receiving in the Complexities of Aging, Illness or Disability*. Woodstock: SkyLight Paths.

Sullivan Burleson, Amy, and Deborah Miller. 2015. "Who Is Taking Care of the Caregiver?" *Journal of Patient Experience* 2, no. 1 (May): 7–12.

Troncoso, Sergio. 1999. "La Abuela." In *The Last Tortilla and Other Stories*, 123–62. Tucson: University of Arizona Press.

CHAPTER 5

Love Comes My Way

YVONNE HURTADO ALLEN

yvonne hurtado allen's essay problematizes the familial ideologies ascribed to adoptee experience. As her life history demonstrates, adoption does not always result in a loving caregiver experience. Loneliness, abandonment, and rejection at times inhibit the bond between the adoptee and their new parents, and the adoptee needs to find other forms of self-care.

Adoption is often seen as an enormous act of love and the ultimate in caregiving. A family takes a child into their home and into their lives, and, it is hoped, the child will grow and thrive, and the new family will bond and be happy. This can be a formal or informal arrangement, and in my family it happened to be both ways. My grandfather's sister was really a cousin who was taken in by his mother when his cousin's sister died. Another relative took in someone else's baby when the mother just left one day, never to be seen again. These relationship changes were apparently seamless, and no one questioned the new child's status in the family. My "aunt," my grandfather's sister, loved my grandfather as her brother her whole life, and even though she knew he wasn't her biological brother, he was and still is known as her brother to all of us. There are some crooked branches in our family tree, but we aren't alone. It happens in many families, even if they don't talk about it.

Placing a child up for adoption is often seen in this society as a selfless act. An often desperate single mother, usually young, usually poor, sends her newborn infant off to a new family who will ostensibly love and nurture the infant into adulthood. They will love it more than if it were from their own bodies because it is a gift, an offering from a woman who denies herself the love of her child for the child's own benefit. At least that is the fairy tale we are sold instead of the many and varied truths of why a child is adopted and not kept, of why an adopted child is not as grateful as the new parents think he or she should be.

Adoption, I have realized, is complex. It seems straightforward and simple enough, and it appears to be successful because it happens all the time and the failures aren't often discussed. Many childless couples are eager for a child to adopt, to have someone to love and be loved by unconditionally. Open adoptions—a more modern invention negotiated between biological and adoptive parents—allow the biological parent to participate in the child's life without the parental responsibility. Closed adoptions do not allow for participation or visitation by, or even divulging the identity of, the biological parents.

Mine was not an open adoption; I doubt there were open adoptions at the time of my adoption. When I petitioned the court to see my real birth certificate in the hope of finding out my father's full name, I was denied twice. Even though I knew his informal name, and I of course knew my mother, I was denied because my petition did not include a reason that the court felt warranted opening the file.

Although legally it was a closed adoption, in practice, it couldn't have been more open. There were no secrets except who my father was. Adoption wasn't all that successful for me, although I preferred it to living with my mother. I knew who my mother was, and I felt unwanted, probably more so than kids who didn't know who their mother was. The hole in my heart wasn't put there by some unknown biological mother I could fantasize about; no, I knew who put it there. I had to adjust, adapt, and become what my grandparents wanted of me in order to survive, in order to stay with them.

I loved my grandmother, but I felt she took me only because she had to. It didn't help that by the time I was a teenager, she was going through menopause, and we fought bitterly until I just gave up and didn't fight anymore. I felt like an orphan. Nobody wanted me. My mother didn't fight for me, and my grandmother didn't want another child to raise. I didn't belong to anyone. I felt alone and like I was nothing.

• • • •

She had a cough for most of the fall, but it wasn't unusual for her, so I was not overly concerned. She had mild respiratory problems for years and was susceptible to pneumonia or bronchitis, especially after a cold in the fall and winter months, when it was chilly and wet in the Pacific Northwest. The cough could, and often did, linger for weeks. But she was still coughing in January, so her doctor decided to schedule an x-ray to see if she had pneumonia. She'd had pneumonia a month or so prior and had taken all her medication, so we all assumed it was gone, but it had lingered. There was something on the x-ray, though, a spot or a suspicious abnormality, so the doctor scheduled her for a scan. She told me about it when we talked during our weekly Friday phone call. "It's probably nothing, but the doctor just wants to make sure, since I have been coughing so much. I'll let you know when I get the results," she said at the end of February.

The next week she called me. She very seldom called me—hardly ever, in fact. I was always the one who called. She said she didn't call because I was always busy; she never knew my schedule or when I would be home, even though I always had Fridays off. She had known that for many years, but she would never acknowledge it so she wouldn't have to call. She didn't think she should have to. It should be me who called her. Weeks could go by, and when I would finally call, she would be pissy and irritated. "Well, I wondered if I was ever going to hear from you again," she would say in her best haughty voice, as if the thought had never occurred to her that she could call me. I didn't think she would actually call; I figured she would wait until Friday, when I usually called her, to tell me the results. But she did call.

All the times I wanted her to call me just once came crashing in, and I wished I could take them all back because I knew whatever she had to say was not going to be good. She called when something bad happened: when my brother died, when my grandfather died, when my grandmother was in surgery, and a few days later, when she died in the hospital. As soon as I heard her voice, I felt the panic in my chest, and I didn't want to hear her say again "I have some bad news." She said it in that voice she used when she was trying to be sweet. She was bad at it, bad at being sweet, but if you heard that voice, it was because she was trying to be compassionate or make you feel better about something, usually something bad, very bad.

"I have stage four lung cancer," my mother said in that voice. That voice that I would never hear again. I don't remember what I said. I don't remember what she said next. I didn't know that would be one of the last times she would be lucid. I didn't know that very soon, she would not know who I was.

I'd started therapy about a year before the call because I thought I needed help to quit smoking, but I ended up healing very old, very deep wounds and becoming a person I had seen glimpses of but could never quite hold on to. My relationship with her had always been rough for me. Maybe for her, too, but I wouldn't know. She kept everything in and hid her life from everyone. You could never really know her; she wouldn't let you in. I loved her, but I was also angry at her. I never thought I was angry at her; I always wanted to be around her, to be like her, to be a part of her. But I was angry. I discovered this in therapy, although I'd probably known it all along. For over half a century I was mad at her: angry that she left me, angry that she never said she was sorry, angry that she never cared how I was. Angry that all my life, I'd had to chase her, had to wait for her attention, had to wonder whether she loved me, had to cater to her or she would sulk. She had to be right every time; there was no arguing with her, and if you dared to defy her, the fire would erupt in her, and she would take you down with her sharp voice and biting words. I never wanted that to befall me, so I didn't cross her. We never argued; I always backed down. But I did bite at her: a nip here, a quick snap there, until she reached her limit and I would back off. I wanted her to hurt, I wanted her to suffer, but she wouldn't. I was just an afterthought, a nuisance that she flicked off like a fly buzzing around her head. I was angry at her, but it was more than that. I was resentful; I was frustrated; I was sad; I missed her; I hated her; I grieved. For her? For me? For the relationship I'd never had—and maybe I didn't really want it, but I wanted the opportunity to have it. I deserved that much. I deserved to have a mother who wanted to be with me. But she didn't.

My grandparents had settled in San Francisco when my mother and aunt were toddlers. They'd moved away from the poverty of a small town in Colorado during the Depression, when they would gather coal that had fallen from the trains along the railroad tracks so they could heat their home. They married young, my grandmother pregnant and ashamed in her off-white wedding dress, and they lived with my grandfather's parents because money was scarce for a musician in rural Colorado.

My grandparents raised me after she got pregnant at fourteen by a boy she barely knew. She'd had sex with him, she said, to get back at my grandmother for checking her sanitary pads to make sure she had a menstrual period every month. She spent most of her pregnancy in a home for pregnant girls, and it only added to her rocky relationship with my grandparents. They favored her sister, my aunt, and they didn't make it a secret. When my grandmother left my grandfather briefly, she took my aunt with her, not my mother, who was younger. She wasn't cared for or cared about, and she knew it. She was defiant, contrary, and bold, and this, this shame and embarrassment of pregnancy, made it worse.

She never talked about it, but when I asked her about it once, she told me about a time she went home for a visit while she was pregnant. Guests showed up unexpectedly, and my grandmother put her in the hall closet until the guests left. She was in the closet for hours while the guests and my grandparents visited, ate food, and had a few drinks. She had to go to the bathroom, and she was tired and hungry, but she stayed in there until the guests left, several hours later. I cried when she told me. I felt guilty for what had happened to her, like it was my fault, but I also cried because it was one time when she actually told me something, confided in me, made me feel important enough to share this experience, horrible as it was. How odd that she chose this experience to share. The object of her embarrassment, her humiliation, her shame was the one she chose to share it with.

When I asked her about the boy, she told me very little about him, my father; she wouldn't even describe what he looked like, although my grandmother had no qualms at all about telling me he was red headed[1] and ugly. I grew up thinking I must be really unlovable and undeserving if my ugly redheaded father didn't want me. She didn't even tell me until I was in my forties that he wasn't ugly and didn't have red hair. She didn't even know his whole name so I could look for him. I accepted that she didn't know his name or his birthday because she was fourteen, and a fourteen-year-old doesn't always know all the vital statistics of a partner. But when I did find him, just a few years ago, I sent her a photo of him at the age she would've known him and asked if it was him. She said she didn't know. "Oh, it could be, I just can't tell," she nonchalantly said as my stomach lurched and my ears stopped hearing.

1. Although there is nothing wrong with red hair, the way my grandmother described it suggested there was.

Tears burning my eyes, I wondered how she could do that to me. After a lifetime of this treatment, I still wondered. If that was true, if she couldn't tell who my biological father was—which I doubted—she could have lied to me. She kept in touch with him after I was born, and he came to see me a few times before my grandmother found out. His parents offered marriage, but my grandmother refused. His face looked just like mine at the same age. She could tell it was him: How could she not? She knew how much I needed to find him, how excited and thrilled I was when I did, and she could have lied. But she didn't. He had already passed when I found him, so what could she have objected to? It crushed me that she wouldn't give me this small thing, this tiny gesture of compassion and care. This tiny bit of love.

After I was born, my grandparents filed the legal documents to adopt me, and she went back to school. My father's family sent him off to another part of the city and a different high school and later to the military. She didn't finish school. She got married and had another child, my half brother. I saw her on and off, occasionally but not on a regular basis. She was in and out of my life for the majority of my childhood. She told me not too long before her diagnosis that she had made me some rompers for summertime when I was a toddler, but I don't remember anything fond or loving from her ever, when I was a child or even later. Nothing motherly, not a loving gesture, no fond memories. She was around, needing financial help from my grandparents, needing rescuing from a bad relationship, needing a babysitter when she went out looking for a new man. Her life was hard—mostly by her own doing, but it was hard. She had five other children; she was mostly a single mother with no job skills, no education, and no child support. She lived in the projects for many years, was on and off welfare for many years, often with bare cupboards and little hope for change. She was around, but not for me.

I longed for her. I would try to stay with her for part of summer vacation, and sometimes she would let me. I stayed for a week or two, and I always felt different because of course, I was. I knew who she was, but she wasn't mine. I often envied the other kids who did live with her, but later I realized she wasn't theirs either. She couldn't be. She couldn't give what had never been given to her.

After my adoption, my grandmother said I was to call my grandparents my parents, and the rest of the family would follow suit. My aunt and my mother would become my sisters, my cousins would be my nieces and nephews, and so on. I accepted it, but nobody else in the family would, so there was much confusion over relationships. But I always knew who she was. The adoption meant nothing to her because nothing changed for her and me. It was the same before and after. I didn't belong to her, and she was fine with that. I never called her anything but *Mrs. A.* for most of my life, and later I just didn't call her anything at all.

I had been with my grandparents since I was born and had always called my grandfather *Daddy*. I called my grandmother *Mama* and my mother *Mommy*, but after the adoption became final when I was about four, that changed. I remember going to the courthouse in my new dress and shoes and being coached by my grandparents on what to say to the judge. After I officially became their daughter, I didn't call my mother *Mommy* anymore, and much later, as an adult, I became uncomfortable calling my grandmother *Mama*.

Adoption comes with some problems, but I was mostly grateful to be adopted. I was grateful because I had seen the way my mother and my siblings lived. My grandmother was strict, but she was home every day from work at six o'clock and never went anywhere without me. She never left me; she never abandoned me. My grandfather was always out of town working, but she never left me. She never really paid much attention to me, but I knew she loved me in some kind of way. She'd adopted me, hadn't she? She kept me around, didn't she? She never left me, did she? I believed my grandparents loved me and wanted the best for me, but they hadn't signed up for a baby fourteen years after their last one. I often felt in the way, a burden, an additional expense they didn't need. I tried to make myself small, invisible; I didn't ask for much and tried to be very, very good. If I wasn't a good girl, what might happen to me? Who would take me? I was unlovable and unwanted, wasn't I? I had to be. So I was obedient and quiet.

Adoption can be a double-edged sword for the child being adopted. At least it was for me. The hole in my heart wasn't like a small-caliber shot that went cleanly through and you could live with, or the neat, bloodless bore of an arrow. It was a big, jagged-edged stab wound, and the knife had been twisted and turned until the wound looked like chopped bloody meat. I didn't know my real father, and my mother didn't want me; my grandparents kept me because they felt obligated, but I could be given away again if I didn't behave. In my little-girl head and heart, I had nobody who really loved me, and I ended up losing my emotions and feelings early on. I hardly ever cried, and I felt very little compassion for others. I couldn't talk about my feelings or even feel them. I was just empty.

I started college twelve years ago at a community college. I originally went because I worked at a job where I encountered many Spanish speakers, and I thought if I could learn some of the language, I would be better at my job. I took Spanish in the evening, and after the second semester, I decided that I should at least finish the AA degree I had started so many years before. I graduated in two years with two degrees and transferred to a university to finish a bachelor's degree in sociology.

During the second year of community college, my daughter came to visit and brought with her the sun that would eventually melt my heart, which had been frozen so many years before. They came for his first birthday and never left. Through the years, my role in his caregiving increased until I became his primary caregiver. My daughter went through many crises and unfortunate traumas that impeded her ability to care for him properly, and instead of doing it badly, she graciously allowed me to care for him until she once again could. Taking care of a toddler as a college student is no easy task, but there was and is nothing I wouldn't do for him. When he would put his chubby dimpled hands on my face and smile, my heart just sang. He loved me unconditionally, and even though my own children love me, this was different, as any grandparent knows. The love is intensified somehow with a grandchild, and with him, with his long curly eyelashes and his soft sweetness, I found my way. My heart slowly began to open, my emotions to return. I cried at movies and commercials. I felt things I never had before. The changes in my life that come from loving and being loved by a small boy with a beautiful heart and long curly eyelashes were and would be immense and profound.

I used to drive up to the Pacific Northwest to see her quite often. She came to see me and my family maybe twice. She came for my older daughter's wedding but didn't stay to visit. She rode the train through a nearby city every year for six or seven years, on her way to visit friends in Southern California, and she didn't stop to see us, not once. She spent weeks with her friends, going to the casino and having fun, but she couldn't stop by. My older daughter moved near me with her two children, and even though my mother had never seen the youngest child, she never stopped here to see her grandchildren or her newest great-grandchild. She never liked kids, she said, especially other people's kids, and she would never babysit my siblings' children. Although she said she loved her grandchildren and great-grandchildren, she never made an effort to see them or even talk to them on the phone.

"Are you still in school? What are you, a professional student? Why is it taking you so long to finish? Are you still at it? I know someone who was getting a PhD, and they are already finished. What do you do there? I have no idea what you are talking about. Oh God, still?" These comments and others I used to hear from her almost weekly about my education. I am the first one in our family to graduate from high school. My people weren't immigrants, but they were poor and lived in farm country. My grandparents went to elementary school. Some of their parents went to school; some didn't. In the mountains and prairies of New Mexico and Colorado, schools were sometimes hard to come by, and only some people went on to high school. My biological parents didn't graduate from high school. But I did. And I graduated from college. She never came to the ceremonies for any of my degrees, nor did she acknowledge the graduation announcements and photos I sent. My grandmother would have been so proud, even if she hadn't known what it was all about. She would have been proud, as she was when I graduated from high school. She had my graduation photo on the wall until she was forced to move out of her house when she was no longer able to live alone, many years after my grandfather died. She used to tell me I could do anything I wanted; I could be anything I wanted to be if I stayed in school. But she could never tell me what *anything* might be.

My youngest sister loves her mother very much. She had a fairly good life with her growing up, as the youngest children usually do. By the time the youngest is born, the parents usually have better jobs and are better at life. She had a better job, a government job, and she was able to live on her own. So my sister had it better than the other kids, and she forgave her for what wasn't good. My sister has a good heart, as they say, a forgiving spirit, and a tolerance for bad behavior, as we were all raised to have. My sister had dancing lessons and her own room. She had more expensive clothes and ate takeout and fast food. She took trips with her dance class and wore expensive costumes and dance shoes.

My sister moved in with our mother and my stepfather several years ago and will stay with her until the end. I call my sister often to check on her own mental health because she is doing this alone. She is watching the time tick down and watching as her mother comes back from chemotherapy, from scans, from treatments, watching as there is less and less in her mother's eyes, less of her to love and to love her. She says her mother is childlike now; she doesn't have responsibilities and doesn't have a short-term memory, and most of the time, the long-term memory is combined with static, so there are parts missing. She doesn't want to take a shower and is pouty and petulant when made to do so.

At other times, however, for the first time in her life, my sister watches her mother be happy. Just happy to be. This is a benefit of the cancer that took over her brain. She no longer hates living in the Pacific Northwest, in the country, afraid of the mountain lions. She no longer hates the snow, the cold, or the gray skies that go on endlessly in winter. She doesn't mind the howling wind or the rolling thunder when the storms come in. She is happy to watch TV, pet the dog, take a nap, and eat. She tried to use the computer again, but she couldn't and just didn't care. She is happy to be. For once in her life, she is happy, and for that I am grateful. She doesn't recognize or remember my sister sometimes, and it hurts my sister horribly, but she understands. I talk to her on the phone, and she doesn't know me most times, but when she does, she doesn't want to talk more than one or two minutes. We used to talk for hours. We used to laugh until she literally wet her pants. We used to sit at the kitchen table drinking coffee in the afternoon. We used to.

I was in therapy for close to a year and went back later for a tune-up. During the tune-up, it was confirmed that I was depressed and anxious and felt my identity slipping away. I had discovered in graduate school that I was old. I know how funny that sounds. I had always felt that I was just a student in school, like everyone else, and for the most part, I was. I felt that I was accepted as just a student, not an old student, an old woman. My friends at school didn't treat me differently, and I only had a couple of professors who didn't treat me the same as other professors did. One gave me a lot of respect and deference, and the other was just uncomfortable around me. But for the most part, I was a student. Even in my semester abroad program, my three roommates and I got along well, and we did many things together, including a trip to Paris. But in graduate school I was no longer just a student. The politics changed, and the resources available went to those who were in the cliques, the little groups of mostly white, mostly middle- or upper-class professors and grad students who were probably the popular mean girls in high school. Scholarships and fellowships are not meant for older students. Programs, internships, jobs on campus are not meant for older students. Professors pick their graduate students early and mentor them, giving them the choice jobs, the benefit of their experience to bring in the fellowships and, later, the postdocs. Theirs are the names on journal articles, on conference roundtables and seminar presentations. They are groomed for the academy, for the research grants, to be the next generation of professors. This is a young person's game, and I, I found out, am not a young person.

I conferred with others who were close to my age or even quite a bit younger and found they, too, had experienced many of the same types of exclusion. I discovered that this place, this institution that I love and hate and that has been my home for many years, is not meant for me. It always tries to get rid of me, to hurt me, to lose me, but I am still here. It hurts, though, and I was shattered. In this way, it reminds me of her.

As a first-generation Latina college student who lived in the projects in East Oakland and went to schools in low-income neighborhoods, I had little of what the university values, so I had a difficult time in college as an older student. Like other students, I was expected to know things I had no idea about, but for me, my age was factored in, and so the expectations were higher. How did I not know how to operate the computer equipment in the classroom? How did I not know how to write a graduate-level paper in the first quarter of my master's program? How did I not know the protocol of the academy? My lack of knowledge in some areas elicited looks of distaste or disgust sometimes from professors or students, and my impostor syndrome skyrocketed. I hoped that I wouldn't be called upon to answer a question, but in grad school, that is the name of the game. You have to be ready every day, and it is a cutthroat competition. The bright young men, especially, need to show off their fancy words and long, overblown explanations. We are enlightened by their expertise, and they cleverly display their talent for memorization as they yammer on, verse after verse, each outdoing the other. I am not a threat to them, and they stare with their heads cocked to the side when I answer a question or take my turn, offering an opinion or interpretation in class when called upon. Then they turn back to each other as if I didn't exist and continue as if I had said nothing.

I would think, How did I get here, anyway? I am not that smart, and others here are so much smarter. They have more knowledge that is valuable here; they fit in better; they speak the same language. I don't belong here.

A few years before I came to the university, my partner and I were driving through town and made a wrong turn. We came upon university housing, and I saw all the bikes in the front and the students walking around, no doubt going to class or the library, getting coffee for a study session. I wondered to myself what it would be like to be a student here, to go to class, to go to the library, to get a coffee for a study session. I never dreamed in my wildest imagination that I would be here. Although I didn't live in university housing, I did do the rest, and I lived my fantasy, my daydream. My love-hate relationship with this place is mostly love. I feel fortunate, blessed, to be here, however unwanted I am.

I went to see a speaker on campus. She'd written a book on impostor syndrome, and the room was filled with young women, many of them Latinas that I knew or had seen before in class or on campus. The room was electric with anticipation that this speaker would have the answers we needed to feel more acceptable, more comfortable, more valuable in this place. But instead of telling us that the institution needed to change, she told us how much and in which ways we needed to change, to adjust, to reframe in order to better suit the academy. We were what was wrong. We weren't impostors so much as we were different and needed to get with the program to succeed.

I'd had my doubts about this woman because although I had heard about impostor syndrome many times, it was worse for women of color, and even worse for older women of color. She was neither. Like a fool, I bought her book anyway, thinking maybe there was some small kernel of wisdom I could take from it in the privacy of my own couch, even though I knew there would not be. I stood in line so she could sign it for me, although I had never heard of her then or since. She asked my name and proceeded to spell it wrong and then asked me how to spell it as if it were something she had never heard of. She messed up my name in the book I bought, and I just couldn't forgive her for it. It was just one more slight, one more way to make me feel small and insignificant. The irony was not lost on me, but I can't think it was irony as much as racist, classist, and intentional. "I saw you at the talk last night. Wasn't she great?" No. No, she wasn't.

She got another scan last week and one more yesterday. The scan of her lungs showed that the cancer has spread and that she has nodules in the lymph nodes and more areas of the lungs. The scan for the brain has not come back yet, but it most likely will be more bad news. She has said she doesn't want the aggressive chemo they will start next week, and the majority of the family thinks her wishes should be honored. Her husband thinks otherwise. My daughter is there now to see her grandmother, probably for the last time. When my grandmother was sick, she thought I was my daughter. She called me by my daughter's name, and I wanted to cry. My mother doesn't know my daughter and doesn't remember my name. The weather will be getting bad, and traveling to her house will soon not be possible, either by air or car.

My first husband was and probably still is a charming man. I met him when I was sixteen years old and very naive and immature in so many ways. Definitely very inexperienced and innocent, although I had already lived through much trauma. I had never really had a real boyfriend before and didn't think I would ever have one because I thought no boy or man would want an ugly girl like me. So the attention he gave me was glorious, and soon I was his.

He turned out to be an abuser of the full-service kind. Physical, emotional, financial, sexual—all of it. It started small and escalated after I moved away to another state with him. I didn't think it was that bad at first. After all, I had seen my aunt with bruises and black eyes from her boyfriends or husbands. I had never seen my mother with bruises, but she did have a broken arm, and I have to think it was her boyfriend who did it.

I found out not too long ago that my grandfather had hit and beat my grandmother after they moved to San Francisco. My grandmother took it for only so long before she left him and did not come back until it was clear that he would never do it again. He didn't. As a matter of fact, the power dynamic changed when she went back to the house, and forever after, she was in charge, and he was never the same. I remember when I was three or four, my grandparents were arguing because he was going out and I remember distinctly her throwing multiple plates at him as he headed for the door. But I didn't relate these things to my own situation. I didn't even realize or recognize the abuse the women in my family endured. It just seemed normal. Everyday activities between men and women.

But I didn't want to live like that. I was scared and miserable. I told my grandmother one day a little bit of what he did, and she told me quite emphatically that I had made my bed and I had to lie in it. Even after she saw it for herself. She helped him hold my head under the bathtub faucet to wash the blood out of a large gash on my head. I had passed out when he threw me to the ground, and my head had been slashed on the corner of the baseboard. After I gained consciousness, she went back home and never spoke of it again. Even though she had gone through it herself and put a stop to it, she let me believe I should take it, that it was my duty to take it. Years later, I talked to my mother about the abuse I was going through, and she said, "Oh, that's too bad, I like [his name]." So I stayed. The two women in my life, the only people I knew to ask for advice, said I should stay with a man who beat me and hurt me in ways that would never be undone. Not only did I have him telling me I was worthless and not fit for anyone else, they were telling me essentially the same thing. I stayed for twelve years before I had the courage to get out with children, no money, nowhere to go, and no plan.

My therapist calls me a miracle. Maybe she says that to everyone, but she said that after all I have gone through, the trauma, the abuse, I was able to change my thinking, my attitude, my worldview, and my life. I was able to get this education and raise my grandson in a completely different way than I raised my own children or the way I was raised. I became a different person.

Looking back, I can see that my childhood set me up to be a target for abusive men. The women in my family were abused in one or more ways—even my great-grandmother, I recently found out. I didn't think I was a part of a pattern of abuse because I wasn't hit by my grandmother. I only thought of abuse in terms of physical abuse and not anything else. I didn't understand that lack of care, lack of attention, and lack of love is also abuse of a child. I subconsciously thought I could get these things from a partner, but I attracted yet another abuser and still lacked the care, attention, and love I didn't know I needed. I spent most of my life walled up, not letting the emotions out or the love in. I thought I was being strong, keeping my hurt tucked away in a box at the back of my mind, not allowing it to affect my life. Of course I was wrong. It affected every part of me and did until recently.

It is said that the best predictor of future behavior is past behavior, but this isn't written in stone and does not mean we are doomed to live as our older generations did. I have been shaped by my family dynamics, of course, but I have had the privilege of an education and therapy to help me stop the cycle of abuse in my family. For me that means more than intimate partner violence; it also means the type of abuse that denies a child love, attention, and care so that they can move upon the earth as a fully feeling, emotionally healthy spiritual being capable of receiving as well as giving love.

Since I originally wrote this, my mother has passed. Quietly in her sleep, as people often do when there is cancer in the brain. She had rallied, and her husband thought she was getting better, that the cancer had gone. I was able to see her during this time, and it was good to see her up and moving around, but she was not there in her head, and I wondered when I looked at her and talked to her what must be going on in her brain when so much of it had been eaten by the cancer that now lived inside her. She was able to understand some things but not others, and I wondered whether she knew she was not the same as she once was. The happiness I had seen in her was gone, as were the drugs, I learned, that had induced it. She was her normal unhappy self, and I felt bad that she couldn't stay in a state of euphoria to the end.

The cancer came back with a vengeance, though, and brought friends. Her back hurt; there was a lump. Her leg hurt. The doctors sent her home with morphine, as there was nothing left for them to do. My sister and stepfather on deathwatch, keeping her as comfortable as possible, my sister giving her chocolate to make her happy. Almost a year and a half after her diagnosis and several months past the eleven months they'd given her to live, just four days after her eighty-second birthday, my sister called me to tell me our mother was gone. I felt very bad for my sister. She took it hard, as I knew that she would. But I didn't cry; I didn't hurt. I didn't see her on the street or in a store, as I had when my brother died so many years ago. I didn't sing her a little song to say goodbye—as I had for my grandfather, alone in the shower after he died—or see her in my dreams.

I felt guilty for not feeling something. I felt like a bad person because I didn't mourn. When people sent their condolences or sympathy, I felt like I didn't deserve them. But I can't help what I don't feel. I can't help that I didn't know her or that she was unable to give what I needed from her. I loved her until I couldn't. I can't help that when I stopped needing her acceptance and love, I was able to see how unhappy and lonely her life was. I can't help but feel sorry for her and for me. The hole in my heart has closed and healed. I found my dad, and although he was already gone, a cousin was able to send me photos and give me some family history, and I found out that he was a good man and a good father to his two sons, my half brothers. He probably would have been a good father to me. The gaping hole left by my mother's abandonment and absence has closed and healed, and although the scars are there, my acceptance of what was has prevented me from judging her more harshly than I have. She didn't care for me for much of my life or take care of me when I needed it, and I have accepted that. I chased a dream of parental love for most of my life, and although it never emerged from the darkness, there was a light that found me.

That light is now twelve years old and hugs me good morning every day. Because of my education and the therapy I was fortunate enough to have, I realized and understood in an almost subconscious way that I had to raise my boy in a different manner than I was raised or than I raised my own children. For so many generations before me, there was violence and dysfunction: children were treated as property and not cherished; partners battled each other because of the pain and suffering of poverty and uncertainty. I had to give my boy better than I got, better than my mother and aunt received, better than my grandparents and great-grandparents received. So raising him is a new experience; it's as if I am a parent for the first time, learning and finding my way with him every day, being careful not to fall into old habits or methods so that he will have a different memory of his childhood than I do, than my children do, than my mother did, than my grandmother did. I work hard for him every day to make sure he feels loved and cherished, respected and wanted, and it is my honor and my great pleasure to be his caretaker.

Adoption can be called the ultimate in caregiving. I could have been adopted by strangers and never have known my family members. But I wasn't. My grandmother decided to adopt me, making it legal that she would be responsible for me until I was eighteen years old. She would be the one to make decisions on my behalf, to teach me what I should know as a child and young adult. She would be the one who would ensure I was healthy and safe. She didn't do a very good job with my mother or my aunt. They both left my grandmother's house at a young age, pregnant and without finishing school. They left with varying traumas and abuse and with stunted cognitive development. They both made the same kinds of mistakes my grandmother made.

I also left my grandmother's house at a young age, but not pregnant, and I did finish high school. My grandmother tried her best, but with generations of bad decisions and bad behaviors, I didn't have much of a chance to be any different from my ancestors. I made bad decisions most of my life. I exhibited bad behaviors most of my life. I almost kept the cycle going, but somehow I have been allowed to stop the cycle, to change the narrative of our family going forward. I was not cared for as a child, but I became a caregiver. To my family, to my students, to my friends. And to me.

CHAPTER 6

Walking the Jagged Edges

Negotiating the Pitfalls of Mental Illness

JOSIE MÉNDEZ-NEGRETE

Josie Méndez-Negrete's paper is an important mentoring resource. The work invites readers to think about all that is done outside of the doctor's office to secure a sustainable life for someone who is often ignored because of the difficulties involved in everyday living. In many ways, Méndez-Negrete is self-taught and indomitable in her care mission. Rather than infantilizing her son, she treats him with respect and refuses the role of the *sufrida* by following her own life path and definition of familial love.

Even if I wanted to put you out of my mind, I can never do that. Good, bad, but never indifferent, you reside in my mind twenty-four seven, where you have permanent residence.

Introduction

After nearly a quarter of a century, it's not unusual for awkward questions to carefully slip from the lips of those who warily ask "How's Tito doing?" Then, a silent gap follows with a shift in conversation, more often than not focusing on my health and asking how I'm feeling. Then, as if by design, be it because of discomfort or shame, the inquisitors move on to things they may have in common with me. Thus, they move from an obligatory greeting that releases them from more intimately learning what it's like to deal with the eternal needs and wants of a son who, because of that dreaded disease, requires my love and care in perpetuity, however long that may last.

Nearly four years after the disease's onset and for more than twenty years, I carried on a long-distance caregiving relationship with the support of family members and the assistance of professionals who barely made do because of cutbacks and defunding to services—my husband was there for me every inch of the way, being my greatest supporter and the best cheerleader for which anyone could ask.

Most recently, for nearly four years and with the support and initiation of my husband, Tito has resided in San Antonio—two and a half years in our home, with the most immediate one and a half years in an assisted living facility—another place in the string of many, with another heavenly name. So, what prepared me to become his mother and take care of him as I have? Or have I done the best I could for Tito?

It's in the Family You Have and Family You Make

By way of an answer, let me offer that throughout my upbringing, I was taught to deal with the complexities of life—all the while not taking anything from anybody, as I have always had the capacity or power to defend myself. To begin with, early in life, I learned to deal with limitations imposed upon me because of gender, as I faced the trauma of emotional pain of abandonment, when Amá immigrated to the United States as a newly approved permanent resident from Tabasco, Zacatecas, Mexico. Until she left, we had been raised in the absence of a father who had contracted himself off as a bracero since before I was born. In that way, my sister and I were spared the trauma of the violence he would dispense upon my mother and middle sister, except for those times he visited the town of our common birth, when he found a way to impose his authority.

As a strategy for the pain and the absence of Amá's presence, my *tía abuela* kept me busy with *artes manuales*, doing embroidery, crocheting, and doll making; reading and writing poetry and short stories; dancing *folklorico* and flamenco; and painting my environment or sketching portraits. These activities became the means by which I learned to cope. The second distraction involved oversight of my mischievous sister, Felisa, who found her own ways to deal with the trauma and pain of Amá's absence. A natural performer, at the cantina that was located catty-corner from Tía Herme's store, Felisa sang and danced for centavos or a soda. At home, my little sister relied on the technology she created to host a cine, showing transparencies of our family photographs and charging a peseta for each viewer. With her shenanigans, Felisa kept us entertained.

I never imagined that these cultural practices would become the balm I relied on to heal the historical trauma and cope with the violence of being an *hija de Juan*, as I fended off the harm and hurts I experienced. Each and every one of the gifts given to me by my great-aunts assisted me to cope with the difficulties of growing up in my father's house and later allayed the stresses and pressures of caregiving for a son with special needs.

Learning to Navigate My Environment

In Tabasco, there were several people perceived as different or strange, but I was taught to see them as people with the right to be in our space and who deserved to be treated honorably. One memory I have is that of a neighbor who lived around the corner from us—she was Sotera's mother—and she was on my path to school: a mentally ill woman who freely and without restraints hurled curses and spit wads in the direction of those who dared walk in front of her house: she had nothing else to do. Restrained in a cage-like structure, this woman gave passersby the thrill of a lifetime. Yet, unlike most of our neighbors, as the bullheaded *cabezona* I knew myself to be, I passed right in front of her house, and, turning in her direction, I gave her *los buenos días*, because she deserved morning greetings and valuation as a human being. My good manners spared me from being a target—in her heart of hearts, she knew I respected her.

Socialization of Difference

There would also be global concerns in my life. The historical trauma embedded in the scars of Spanish colonization and Yankee imperialism, as Tío Pepe would often remind me, framed notions of my social position, as I learned that the structural inequalities with which I dealt were not all carved in my Mexican upbringing. Up to that time, our economic class had been irrelevant, as the two of us who were left behind—my sister and me—lived under the illusion of wealth because of the nearly thirteen dollars a month we received in remittances, which our parents sent from Weslaco, Texas. For those three years of Amá's absence, Felisa and I had all the comforts of home, with new toys and dresses when we wished. It did not take long before we adapted and thrived in the care of our great-aunts.

Race and ethnicity were nonissues in my growing-up years and would become concerns only when we migrated, even though we partook in expressing anti-Indigenous sentiments that pervaded the vernacular of the town—colluding with notions that *los huicholes* and gitanos were *robachicos*, while *indios* were *pata rajadas*, or those who wore a nopal cactus on their forehead—as a way to ethnically deride them, taking sides with the criollos in power. When I was eleven and Felisa merely five and without documents, we joined our family in *el norte*. We were without documents because my parents lacked the $1,500 bond per child, for a total of $3,000, for us to legally immigrate. In our hometown, the microaggressions we experienced were limited to insults about being parentless when our parents chose el norte over us.

Still, once in the United States, while we were spared racialization, instead, internalized racism, ethnocentrism, and classism would become the wedge that kept my peers at a distance from me. We were silenced in our heritage language because Spanish was prohibited in school, so my initial six months of education were those of an academic mute—no one spoke to me. However, in those days when a sink-or-swim approach to English was preferred, dictionaries and books bridged my acquisition of a second language. Books became my shelter. And my creative expressions—which were now limited to making rag dolls from the leftover pieces of material in Amá's sewing basket, as well as sketching and drawing—became my means to cope with the violent home and the madman who was our father, as I now lacked access to the creative resources previously available to me.

It was then that writing poetry and short stories and keeping a journal became my own way of documenting the world, however gray and depressing it was. Still, I found the time to draw portraits of the Beatles, which I sold to those who longed to collect their favorite musician from my stash. In my long string of writings, one of the short stories that I initially created for English 1A at San José City College became the writing sample I would submit for my doctoral application at the University of California, Santa Cruz. As I recall memories of my childhood and youth, I remember that I read some poems in our local community and at our Mexican cultural celebrations.

A fortunate person, despite a spotty and suspect education because of my legal status, as a graduate student at the University of California, Santa Cruz, I was introduced to theoretical points of departure that gave me the language to place in context what I was attempting to understand, as I examined multiple forms of violence in our family, and in my trajectory as a nontraditional student who returned to school to complete a PhD after having received a master's of social work from San José State University.

It was higher education that allowed me to further explore my life experience to tell stories that many carry, as I shed the pain and the shame and broke the silence. As a sociologist, I had long pondered material and historical conditions that framed family abuse; it was sociological thought that allowed me to begin examining family and community interactions and create meaning in the context of my lived experiences—symbolic interactionism, emotion management, and notions of daily relational interactions served me well.

On Becoming a Mother

Those early years of my childhood, I never imagined having children, although I thought about joining a convent to make a difference in the lives of women and children—I was always one who wanted to change the world and improve the lives of others.

In school, I would learn about fertilization and the birthing process, but that was about the extent of education related to anything carnal. Later, at a premarital exam, I was informed I had a severely tilted uterus that would keep me from having children. So when the children I was not supposed to have arrived, I had no clue regarding the dance of life I would engage in with them, except for the desire to not hurt them. So, I assessed their exterior appearance to evaluate their well-being. Does he have all his limbs? Can he see? Can he hear? Does he follow your finger with his eyes? Does he recognize your voice? Is he voiding his body fluids properly? Careful *que no se le caiga la mollera*, or make sure he doesn't fall on the soft spot on his head because the child will have problems later.

As a mother, my main concern became my children's basic needs. Still, I entered motherhood with notions that they would not experience the physical, psychological, emotional, or spiritual wounding I had survived; as the firstborn child of my home, I had sworn never to enact brutality on my children. Alternative disciplinary measures became the norm in my family. Among the strategies I relied upon were warnings, counting from one to five for grave offenses, or taking away privileges and toys that they especially enjoyed—but never hitting them. Never in my imagination did I envision becoming a caregiver for life, especially in the individualist society into which my children were born—normative expectations being that they move out on their own at the age of eighteen. While Tito moved out before eighteen to live in the home of his girlfriend, it was not to become independent. A couple of years into that journey, our mother-son relationship became more complex with the onset of mental illness three months before Tito turned twenty-one.

Life Goes On: Caregiver and Mother for Life

It was thus that I became Don Quixote to my son's Sancho Panza, as we dealt with his health and the institutions became the windmills with which we would contend. Mental facilities rejected him, diagnosing Tito as a druggie who was not mentally ill, and drug recovery programs refused him services because he was in need of mental health treatment, with the excuse that he required more than they could do for him.

Without options, I sought out the support of an Indigenous healer, thinking he would at least be able to point us in the direction of alternative means. However useful this was, it took almost three years to finally find a group of service providers—a recently funded dual-diagnosis program had started in San José, California—who were researchers interested in understanding the self-medication process of drug use for those who are mentally ill and rely on drugs to normalize their conditions. Before that, feeling empathy for both of us, a religious recovery group that went by the name Victory Outreach accepted him into their program, but he soon bolted from the facility. Thus, Tito reached his entry point into the world of mental illness facilities.

Prior to his in-and-out existence in mental health care, Tito lived with me in Santa Cruz, California, while my husband worked as a postdoc at the University of California, San Francisco. Even though Tito's diagnosis came with all the "positive" conditions of schizophrenia—paranoia, delusions, and gustatory and auditory hallucinations—his mind sped through the stories he carried as his mind evolved the psychosis that rooted in him. My husband included him in our outings when I traveled to San Francisco or when my husband came to Santa Cruz, where he found things for Tito to do.

As I had been advanced to candidacy in my PhD program, I was able to be there for Tito. Thus, I tended to his basic needs—I cooked, cleaned, and listened to him—albeit not always willingly, as I kept intermittent meetings with my academic adviser. With his fear so deep, Tito attached himself to me, often interrupting my work and expressing the need to speak and be heard. I made my best effort to stop and listen but continued to transcribe, analyze, and write the narrative for my dissertation; work became another coping mechanism by which I could escape my reality. It was difficult to give him my undivided attention, and that was what he felt he needed and was what he demanded. Yet his clinginess and dependency intensified. Then, with Tito's consent, I began to search for a residential facility into which he could move so I could continue doing my academic work.

That move was the most difficult for me. I was accused of abandoning him and judged as an unfit mother, even though Tito was over the age of twenty-one—in my family's eyes, I was doing it all wrong. With compassion and acceptance, my sister Felisa was there for me. Meanwhile, some of my siblings pushed Tito away; as they reminded me, Tito was my responsibility, and they urged me to stop my academic work, almost commanding me to tend to Tito's needs: "Stop and take care of him; he's your responsibility, you're his mother."

His first flight into health, when he tried to run away from his illness, Tito left for Sacramento, hitching a ride with an alcoholic who drove drunk, and ended up at the hospital as a result of an accident. He would later say that felt that if he left the area or place where he lived, things would improve for him. My middle sister received Tito at her home but called me to tell me she could not allow him to stay and had her husband drive him to San José, where I took him to Emergency Psychiatric Services—he was in desperate need of being assessed. After much advocacy, Emergency Psychiatric Services accepted him for evaluation.

Throughout his illness, some relatives and friends have distanced themselves from him, in fear that he could harm them or their children, relying on all the stereotypes society has dispensed about mentally ill people. Through all this, meditation, prayer, and imagination—creative as well as academic writing—has kept me afloat. Within my immediate, long-distance, and near-distance relationship with Tito, I have not hidden my family dynamics as

I completed the dissertation; I have been open about having a child with special needs and have never used him as an excuse for failing to complete my work. Thankfully, because I've worked as a social worker, former students and professional colleagues became part of my support network. The gifts I had been given by my great-aunts also became another means by which I kept myself afloat amid the needs and wants expressed by my son.

If it were not for the support of those friends that continue to be members of my chosen social family, Felisa, my sister, who co-mothered with me from a distance, and the professional and support people who worked with him, who have helped him on his journey, I would have not been able to deal with and cope with the consequences of the illness with which my son deals. Also, Amá always created a space and cooked for him at least once a week. Among the many places in which Tito resided, he found service providers, girlfriends, and friends who allowed him to have a social life, so as not to fall in the pit of the clinical depression also associated with the disease. In addition to those in my family, all those who supported Tito—Lorelei, Belinda and Gilbert, Michael, and Elisa—made my son feel loved and supported.

All these friends and family members made it possible for me to succeed in my profession and to reach full professor status by writing two books and countless articles that I could not have written without their support. It was the almost-two-thousand-mile distance, from California to Texas, that created the space to do the work I did. With their support, I was able to set limits and accept that I could only do what I could and that Tito had to learn to deal with the illness as he relied on and learned to accept resources at his disposal to live his life as best he could. The distances taught me to let go without abandoning him. I gave myself permission to understand the disease and the ways in which it affected each and every one of us, whether we maintained contact with Tito or not. I let go of the guilt and embraced the child who was born to me, with the understanding that he and I have come into each other's lives to learn from one another and become the best human beings possible.

Our journey has been and continues to be an arduous path. Countless flights into health (running away from the illness, not the system); suicidal talk; the consequences and side effects of the neuroleptics and psychotropic medications Tito takes—diabetes being the worst. Tito finally recognizes that the medicine make him better able to deal with the disease. With time, Tito has become a mentor and supporter of those who are mentally ill; he tells them his story and helps them understand the value of the medication and the benefits of taking the prescribed doses, as he shares coping strategies he uses when life becomes difficult to bear.

The Beginning and the End

It was a cold Christmas Eve, December 24, 2014, in San José, California. My forty-something son, Tito, expected my husband and me to arrive for the holidays. With an amazing psychic connection, it was not more than five minutes after parking the car and bringing in our luggage that the telephone rang. The urgency in my son's voice was so palpable it shattered my heart.

> Momma, I can't stand to live under this condition. I'm sick and tired of it, and if you don't take me out of here, I'm going to kill myself. [Brief pause.] You have no idea, in this independent living house I have been assigned to an incontinent man who runs at both ends—he urinates and defecates at all hours of the day. There's no one to clean up after him. I have to clean him and wash my own stuff that he soils . . . blankets, clothes, walls. Come take me home. I don't wanna be here anymore.
>
> Tito, Christmas Eve 2014

This twenty-plus-year journey was something I never imagined traversing. When my son, Tito, was first diagnosed with mental illness sometime in the early 1990s, I reviewed my family's medical legacy—on both paternal and maternal sides—to find a genetic origin for the disease in our family history. My mother became my first point of contact, and because she knew our history on our paternal side, I was able to learn that my paternal great-grandfather had lived with epilepsy and that when my father went to prison, he was diagnosed as a sociopath. No one on my maternal side was identified as strange or as a loco—the term that would have been used.

Then, I examined myself—what I ate, what illnesses I might have had the first trimester of pregnancy (a cold or a flu, for example), and what I ate that might have affected my pregnancy. Somehow, I had to rule out his condition being my fault, and having read that genetics may be implicated and also understanding that environment contributes to the onset of the disease, I began to examine my treatment of Tito and how I might have brought about his condition. Soon enough, after I had explored all the possibilities, he and I began to search for ways in which he could be helped or get support.

But our journey continues, and not without its complications. In our naivete, my husband and I brought Tito to San Antonio, Texas, without having any options for his treatment, albeit with a prescription that would give him medications for three months. Long-distance care was like an itinerant vacation where I went to visit family and friends as I checked up on Tito wherever he happened to reside.

Before long, Tito became my twenty-four-seven responsibility. I was thankful for my professional preparation. As a social worker who had learned about the resources available and who had taught graduate students to secure resources and advocate for those in need, I began the process of securing a primary doctor and a psychiatrist with the expectation that Tito would reside in our home.

As a family, we quickly learned the ways in which, as a formerly institutionalized man, he had developed oppositional patterns: he found ways to do what he wanted, when he wanted, because he was his own person, and no one was going to tell him what to do. After all, he was an adult who knew what was best for him. But that was often doubtful—he drank more sodas than I would have allowed, but smoked less than before because his dad put him on a one-pack limit that he honored because his dad said so.

My husband and I agreed that he was an adult and his own person. However, we reminded him that he lived in a household with other adults who had responsibility to the home as well as to each other. And we tried to get him to honor a schedule, to take his pills on time, to eat healthily, and to reduce his smoking and soda intake. Those were not difficult requests to monitor, as I purchased and dispensed the cigarettes and the sodas per an agreement with him. For the most part, that was an easy bridge to cross. Soon, other difficulties surfaced. Those demands and conditions that I could manage from afar—mostly by giving in to him or figuring out a way to get his wants met, through Felisa as an intermediary—created more conflict, front and center.

As his representative payee, I assumed responsibility for his income, which was less than $1,000 a month. He lacked the notion of money and wanted it when he asked for it because he had it, as he saw it. Finances became a serious point of contention for Tito and me. More difficult than his constant need for money, which he often thought I was taking from him and using for other purposes, was the intermittent psychosis that would overtake him, which became more intense with the stresses and loneliness of living in a home with two professionals who assumed and carried out their duties in a responsible way. The loneliness and isolation became points of distress for Tito. Thus, in addition to still attempting to secure remedial and psychiatric resources in a town with very limited services, as the primary caregiver, I found myself working out of the home so that he would not be alone in it.

With his urinary incontinency as a problem, our home became an uncomfortable place because of the stench; we tried antiodor sprays and soon had to replace the bed in which he slept, as he continued to refuse to wear adult diapers at night to protect the bedding and the mattress. Finally, I secured a medical doctor and a psychiatrist. I took him to all his appointments and his blood draws, as they had to monitor the medication he was prescribed. I went to all these appointments and inserted myself in them, and with a release from him that allowed me to be a part of his appointments, I was able to ask questions and provide additional information about his well-being without being intrusive, and in as supportive a way as possible, I contributed to his treatment. Yet his life conditions would also create chaos in my own body and health.

In Reciprocity—His Illness Is My Illness

Tito would not be the only one who would deal with the disease—depression would hover over me, and to abate its impact I began walking and doing exercise, as well as monitoring what I ate, using portion control as a way to lose weight and monitor my health. Woven into my profession was the creation of art, as I continued to sew, paint, and draw images that cleared my psyche and allowed me to see the beauty in life.

The stress and pressure of taking care of Tito led to diabetes, a disease that I refused to acknowledge, even though I researched alternative ways to heal myself, beginning with diet. I increased my intake of nopales and other greens such as verdolagas and okra, along with medicinal teas. For about three years, I was in denial.

Finally, after realizing that I was harming my body, I went to the doctor, who informed me I was borderline diabetic but told me that I could do exercise and fend it off with diet. So I took his advice and continued to learn better ways of taking care of myself, as I relearned to love myself. With the constant stress and pressure of my caregiving responsibilities, there was no turning back: the doctor diagnosed high blood pressure and cholesterol problems, and I was placed on medication—three different types.

More committed to exercise and keeping a diet that helped me deal with diabetes, I lost more than forty pounds, without restricting my diet but by monitoring the food that was most likely to hurt me. When he lived in our home, Tito had become a self-appointed meds monitor and often asked me or reminded me to take my pills, telling me to not stray from taking them because I needed the medicine to stay healthy. After a good morning greeting, he would ask me if I had taken my medicine, and he still does this when he comes to breakfast on Saturday or Sunday, depending on our schedule. As he became an ally in my health, he learned to access resources for his health as he navigated the city.

Before long, with a bus pass in hand, Tito learned the lay of the land and traveled to all parts of San Antonio. He volunteered in a couple of community organizations, participated in a social support group, and found himself a day treatment that allowed him to create a network of friends. Rather than becoming comfortable with each other, our situation became tense, and both he and I became depressed with the situation. Before the sixth of every month, when his income would be automatically deposited at the bank, he would ask for his money so he could live an independent life, as he imagined it.

Because I did not see this as a positive step for him, I refused to give him the money and told him he could continue to live in our house so long as he cooperated and followed the rules that all of us in the household maintained. He continued to try. The stress was wearing on him and me. He had done some research on moving, looking around and visiting places as well as talking to some of his peers with whom he attended day treatment. The day came when he asked to move out.

"Momma, I'm going to go crazy if I don't move. I've found a place near here. Can we go look at it?"

By July 11, 2017, Tito had found a new home. It was a residential facility where they would administer his medication, provide room and board, and take him to all his doctors' appointments. It's less than a mile from our home. The protection of that distance for both Tito and me created the comfort and healing space we both needed to move on with our lives. In his new environment, other problems would arise—he'd fear that the residents would rape or abuse him, for example. Soon other scenes of psychosis and the delusions and hallucinations would emerge.

He now calls the place in which he lives "home." Still, every so often he wants to leave the facility, often telling me that I "betrayed" him because he went to live in an institution rather than stay home with us. I do not argue that point but assert that he is where he is best attended to and that the resources are limited, and I do not want him in a board-and-care home where they will do very little and badly nourish him for the limited resources he has. Sometimes he agrees. Other times he accuses me of stealing from him.

Sometime early this year, 2018, Tito called asking me to listen to him. Soon, he refused to speak because "they are listening." He once again expressed that he is not safe where he lives—drugs, alcohol, and his treatment by the residents were his points of contention. He added that "I want my money, and I don't want to live here." And "If you don't give me my money, I am going to send you to prison for stealing my money." When he couldn't move me, he hurled personal attacks. "You're evil" and "You have no heart" were but some of the complaints he blurted out. From there he asked for something to eat and coffee to drink. I asked him to walk over and said I would feed him. When he arrived, his script had changed:

"I want to go to SAC [San Antonio College] to enroll in school. Drop me off in the morning. Why do you help your students when you don't even want to bother with me?"

More often than not, if Tito is experiencing a psychotic break of whatever degree, I do not call the director of the place in which he resides. However, this time I did because he felt so unsafe, he was shaking when he told me.

It is the end of October 2018, and Tito has had two good weeks. The incessant calls have become almost silent; he has displayed a loving and caring attitude, greeting me each morning, expressing hope for the day. Still, he is feeling depressed because he turned down a busboy job he was offered. He feared failing or experiencing difficulty and chose to not show up, taking confidence in the three-day job he has at a friend's gallery; "It's not much money but provides me with spending money and provides me change above and beyond the allowance you give me." He is doing the best he can with what is available to him, although he is not content with his lot in life. He is ambitious and imaginative, but the passion he needs to make something happen for himself is not there—school, work, and other interests are but part of the kaleidoscope of his imaginary world, which opens up as well as restricts whatever options he imagines for himself.

Coping Skills and Dealing with Mental Illness

I have my disease under control. At my most recent doctor's visit, all my numbers were good, and there was no problem with my urine. My body is strong, and I have to speed up my exercise routine. Mindfully, I have to keep myself strong so that I may be there for Tito.

As I continue to stay healthy, I am feeling thankful and hopeful. Yet the reality of the unpredictable disease with which Tito has lived for about a quarter of a century keeps me on my toes—it is one day at a time for us. Our path is not easy, but the lessons learned for him and me will continue to be diamonds in the rough. With my husband's support, we have arrived at a place of hope. Also, with his help I have learned to see and understand that Tito's life will shift from coping to chaos and that I must be there to help him with what I am able to carry, without doing it for him, but supporting him in the process. Without my husband's support, insight, and love, it would be extremely difficult to deal with Tito's needs. But, like Tito, every day I wake up open to the possibilities as I get ready for another day with him, to do the best I can with what I have.

Still, there are lessons to glean from our lived experiences. To keep my sanity and support him the process, I must remember the following:

- Dump the shame, responsibility, and regret for what was and could have been—it is what it is; deal with it the best you can.
- The disease is not Tito's or my fault.
- Love him as he is and be there with appropriate limits.
- Accept that he has all he needs and that he is living a more fulfilled life since he moved "home" to San Antonio.
- Rest on the reality that chaos and uncertainty are central in his life and in ours.
- Recognize and follow through with the knowledge that I cannot give him everything he wants.
- Remember that giving in to him only results in his asking for or wanting more.

- My "no" is self-protection and self-preservation. Be okay with using it in kindness.
- The more authentic, honest, and firm I am, the better able I will be to relate with him, and the better we will cope with each other.

I recognize that my son is loving, compassionate, brilliant, and giving. It is my wish for him to have the life he aspires to have and for him to find the companion he thinks he needs in order to be happy. Most of all, I want Tito to embrace self-love and to be okay with who he is; he has given much and has tested me much. Still, I would not replace him with a perfect specimen of a human—he is my dearest Tito, and I love him as he is. Nonetheless, with our parallel illnesses, we need to do all we can to tend to our bodies, minds, and spirits.

CHAPTER 7

Chronicle of a Caregiver

A False Notion of Autonomy

ENRIQUETA VALDEZ-CURIEL

Enriqueta Valdez-Curiel's essay draws attention to the transnational aspect of caregiving across the U.S.-Mexico border as well as the role of family members who are clinicians and caregiver advocates and who possess special insider's knowledge due to their double positionality.

I am fifty-seven years old. I never had children, nor did I want to have them. I was never married, nor did I care to be married. I always saw myself as free with no one to take care of. I thought that no one—apart from myself—would take care of me. Once I had two cats. I loved them madly, but after eighteen years of being with me, when they died, I felt freed from the responsibility of caring for them. I was convinced that I would never follow traditional gender-role patterns of most Latinas (Zambrana 1995), especially those providing unpaid care.

As a child, I lived with my grandparents for many years, watching my grandmother caring for my grandfather and his chronic illnesses. Later, I watched Mamita caring for my father when he was ill—and I call her Mamita because I love her so very much, but don't misunderstand me: she's very strong; she's never been fragile. However, I never observed women in the family taking care of their mothers, nor men taking care of wives.

Remaining single and childless would—I assumed—free me from the cultural script of *marianismo* (Mendez-Luck and Anthony 2016; Englander, Yanez, and Barney 2012), familism (Flores et al. 2009), and intergenerational caregiving roles (Williams et al. 2014) in my Latino/a family. My concept of feminism tolerates no place for the traditional role of caregiver. Therefore, I never saw myself, my work, my travel, and my free time limited by the need to provide caregiving.

Sometimes when we are young, we think our parents will spend the rest of their lives in their fifties—strong and healthy, waiting just a few more years for peaceful retirement. We cannot conceive that in the future they will be tired and old, with ailments inherent to age. It never crosses our minds that one day caregiving roles will be reversed and our parents will turn to us for care. Or we realize it is our turn to care for them. If not us, then who will do it?

I was fifty-three years of age and Mamita seventy-nine when I realized that being a *single*, childless doctor with a flexible job made me, according to our culture, the perfect kinship-caregiver. Were not all those variables supposed to free me from that traditional role? My whole plan worked in reverse, and here I chronicle my journey of how I became an almost perfect Latina kinship-caregiver to a dependent adult.

What happened next was the very thing that I always feared would happen. Mama carried a lot of bitterness within herself. I knew it was very likely that her gastrointestinal discomfort, stress, and hatred would eat her up inside, would oxidize her own cells (Soung and Kim 2015), leading her to develop some illness inside. Her difficult life with my father obsessed her, waking and sleeping. Sometimes she even dreamed that she screamed at him, which woke her up sweating with fear.

My father died April 17, 2001, but today, the memory of his words still haunts and harms us from afar. Every time Mama remembers him—and it is unusual for a day to pass that she fails to remember—her voice sounds raspy with rage, discrete lines turn her forehead into furrows, and three small vertical lines narrow the distance between her brows. At that moment, I know that adrenaline accelerates her heartbeat and blood surges through her vessels hurled along by the cursed memories. In those moments, I am distressed, too, because I know that all this turmoil harms my mother in a way she herself is unaware of.

These are what I call "accursed memories," since they represent an imprecatory curse. Her painful memories of life with my father are so powerful that they invoked a curse upon my mother and me. I undergo suffering with her. She lives with great pain, anger, and regret that she stayed with him all those miserable years. She cannot change her past. She cannot forget it.

When Mama remembers my father, anger rises in her as she *echa pestes* (throws curses) against him. She would like him to come back to life to tell him all she has to say that burns inside of her, but that caustic desire itself inflames her soul and the interior of her body. Her thoughts consume her and consume me with her: I feel that I also pay the consequences of such emotional damage since I, as a kinship-caregiver, accompany her to take care of her illnesses.

For me as a caregiver to reduce our stress, I needed Mama to try to come to terms with her past. Neither she nor I can change it, and we both deserve peace. Before Mamita could move toward tranquility, however, what I feared most came to pass.

News of my mother's cancer arrived in December 2017, while we were living in Mexico. We were never free of the augury of things to come, always enveloping us. Throughout Mama's life, the organs of her digestive system took turns presenting the discomfort reflected by the desecrated environment surrounding her family life and her work in the fields of California. Mamita arrived at age seventy-eight accompanied by many alarming signs and symptoms of gastrointestinal discomfort: chronic constipation, gastric reflux, blood in the stool, anemia, weight loss, pain, and a *bola* (ball) *debajo de la costilla derecha* (under the right side of her rib). As she mentioned the bola, she pointed under her rib on the right and complained of *flojera* (laziness), *mucha, mucha flojera!* In medical terms we translate *flojera* as fatigue.

Such laziness is opposed to the dynamic character of my mother. Mama is—and has always been—a very strong, tireless worker. However, when she feels tired or weak, she calls herself "lazy," but this word is misleading. She has never been lazy. What she experienced was weakness and exhaustion, medically recognized as asthenia, and in her case, the result of cancer and severe anemia.

All these collected signs and symptoms correspond to colon cancer (DeVita, Lawrence, and Rosenberg 2016), but when we arrived in California, we still had no biopsy of what her private gastroenterologist in Mexico and I thought was a colon tumor. The biopsy represents the necessary, sufficient, and accurate evidence that validates the signs and symptoms of colon cancer. Mama's colon was so inflamed when we were in Mexico, it was impossible to reach the tumor area through the colonoscopy. Faced with failure to perform the biopsy, the gastroenterologist requested a search for tumor markers in the blood. Her doctor ordered a blood test to search for carcinoembryonic antigen and cancer antigen 19-9, markers secreted by colon cancer tumor cells. All markers were in their normal ranges, giving us some hope that the bola that Mama touched debajo de la costilla was benign.

However, tumor markers sometimes give false negatives, and the omen that this was the case with my mother's tumor marker was almost obvious because she had characteristic signs of colon cancer: change in bowel habits, bloating, blood in the stool, anemia, weakness, fatigue, and weight loss. For this reason, tumor markers are valid for diagnosis only when they are accompanied by other tests, such as a colonoscopy. In medicine, the false negative denies the presence of abnormal change or disease when it exists. Therefore, the false negative is considered an error. Similar to medical results, we also encounter false negatives as metaphors in life.

For example, before they married, my father *enamoró* (made my mother fall in love with him) with false words. He claimed, "I would never mistreat a woman. I would never hit a woman, not even with a finger. I would never disrespect a woman with bad words." To her, he seemed so unlike most rural men she knew. Therefore, she thought, Ah, here is the perfect man for me! He made her believe that he was incapable of mistreating a woman, but tragically, metaphorically, literally, he turned out to be a false negative. He devoted himself and his life to mistreating her.

Given our suspicion of colon cancer, with the impossibility of taking a biopsy through the colonoscopy and given tumor markers that contradicted what my mother's body *decía a gritos* (shouted at us), the only option left to confirm the diagnosis was to take a biopsy during surgery. That is, to perform surgery to reach the tumor, take the biopsy, and analyze it immediately to decide how to proceed in the operating room based on results of the biopsy.

As I am narrating it now, with simpler words and with a very patient and hopeful tone in my voice, I always honestly explained all this to Mama, even before the doctors spoke to her. Thus, when we were in the doctor's office, the technical and sometimes confusing language that doctors use only validated what her daughter (also a doctor) had already told her. While I explained all these medical terms in words she understood that did not alarm her beyond reality, I wondered, How would families lacking doctors or nurses among friends or relatives resolve these doubts and fears during health crises?

Physicians are required to inform patients about diagnoses, prognoses, and possible palliative and preventive care, but information must be dispensed with appropriate, sensitive cultural regard. Such strategic, critical communication is a plus—and I would say a luxury—often absent in medical practice. Perhaps this is the reason why in Mexico we say that every family must contain a doctor and a lawyer. I agree. Without my medical training and expertise, it would be difficult to understand what was happening to Mama and how to become her caregiver appropriately.

To return to the urgent need for a biopsy, her Mexican gastroenterologist and I were sure she would require surgery because the tumor already obstructed her intestine. If we opted for surgery to take place in Mexico, it would have to go through the Mexican Social Security Institute, which pays for health insurance there and would cover all her medical expenses.

However, this option implied months of waiting, since the Mexican Social Security Institute has an excessive demand for surgeries, and in general, a constant demand to treat patients in all services far beyond its capacities. Thus, we consulted a private gastroenterologist. Waiting for months to determine whether the tumor was benign or malignant could make the difference between life or death. A second option was to select a private medical service in Mexico, but the high costs of surgery and possible chemotherapy were beyond our means. That was when we looked to *el norte* (the north), to go to California, where Mamita lived, worked, and retired, entitling her to Medicare and Medi-Cal health services.

Although we were unfamiliar with California's health care system, since Mama rarely used it, as a doctor I knew that the required referral procedure would delay us. In California, we started our medical journey in the emergency room (ER). Armed with all the medical evidence from Mexico and knowing that no one can be denied treatment in the ER, we avoided protocols requiring patients to start with a referral from a family physician.

Mama was registered with Social Security as a resident of Salinas, California, but I investigated whether the hospital in Salinas or in Davis, California, offered faster access to medical services. Considering the higher population density of Salinas, moving Mama's residence to Davis offered many advantages for medical procedures. Medical services at the hospital in Davis—compared to the hospital in Salinas—would be faster. Besides, I knew that if we had primary health providers in Davis, Mama would be sent to Sacramento for surgery. I was sure that Sacramento, California's state capital, must provide excellent medical services because politicians who often work there would demand the best services. Yes, I had to consider all these variables—and even many more.

From Mexico, we arrived in Davis, where a friend offered housing and a car. The next day we went to the ER at the local not-for-profit hospital. Yolo County honored Mama's request to change her residence from Monterey to Yolo County. Pondering population density and community economic status are strategies not every family caregiver considers. I know public health and its reality. Unfortunately, the quality of health services varies depending on the region.

Based on the complaint "abdominal pain and intestinal bleeding," immediately we were admitted to the ER. With abdominal pain present day and night, Mama was still bleeding. With the blood tests administered in Mexico—complete blood count, liver enzymes, tumor marker, and the computed tomography (CT) scan showing the tumor—there was no reason to deny or to delay her case for the referral protocol to a specialist. Kinship-caregivers may be unaware of or ignore these facts.

The ER doctor evaluated Mama by interpreting the CT scan. During this assessment I acted as the translator. When he gave his diagnosis, he looked only at me. Perhaps the doctor assumed that she did not understand the English language. He blurted out his diagnosis in front of her, failing to address her as his patient: "*Your mother has cancer*."

You should never assume that patients who ask for a translator fail to understand English—they may feel insecure and uncomfortable in speaking. He was imprudent. Mama understands, speaks, and writes English, but in a medical environment, she feels much more comfortable and confident if I speak for her, a service Latino/a children frequently do for parents as part of our invisible caregiving tasks. Providers often make this common, arrogant, hasty conclusion.

I was indignant. He was thoughtless. It was an insult to jump to a diagnosis without necessary and sufficient evidence. The shockwave of his words swept over my body as if I had entered a cloud of liquid helium. That Mamita had cancer took me by no surprise, nor did it paralyze me. I had suspected that her tumor was cancerous; the urgency of surgical and chemotherapeutical interventions sped us to California. When the ER doctor gave me the diagnosis so coldly, ignoring his patient, his behavior baffled me. Without certainty, without evidence of cancer cells, no medical professional has the right to diagnose cancer.

In 1994 Mama had retired from working on the assembly line in Salinas, California, for Dole Food Company. After over forty-five years living and working in California, she returned to Mexico never intending to live in a country other than the one of her birth. Since then, her infrequent trips to California were always to visit friends or to travel as a tourist—and as the proverb says, *Uno pone y Dios dispone* (Man proposes but God disposes). After almost two decades of retirement in Mexico, sudden alarming symptoms forced her to return to el norte with all the uncertainty of not knowing how long she would be here.

At the doctor's pronouncement Mama anxiously turned to me to ask, "Does he say that I do have cancer?" I could not lie to her. She understood everything he said perfectly.

I answered in anguish: "He cannot say for sure, Mama. We will know only after the biopsy is done. Pay no attention to him. The important thing is that he will refer us to a gastroenterologist who can do the colonoscopy and the biopsy as soon as possible. Then, and only then, will we know what you have."

As a medical student, and now as a doctor and professor teaching future doctors, I always favor respecting the rights of patients to know their diagnoses. Ethically and legally, under the patient's autonomy, the patient has the right to know the diagnosis and prognosis. This critical information is never to be hidden, nor is it ever to be conveyed first to others (Fallowfield, Jenkins, and Beveridge 2002; Jensen and Mooney 1990; Katz 1986; McCabe, Wood, and Goldberg 2010). I share with Katz (1986) the ethical belief that hiding the diagnosis from a patient denies them their right to decide and goes against their dignity.

However, the ethics of the doctor-patient relationship are well established as "principles of beneficence and non-maleficence" giving physicians the possibility to consider the educational, familial, and cultural circumstances of each patient. Physicians must find the best moment or best way to communicate information that can change a patient's daily routine or the rest of the patient's life (Beauchamp and Childress 1994; Hallenbeck and Arnold 2007; Jotkowitz, Glick, and Gesundheit 2006). In our case, the emergency doctor was not only patronizing in judging my mother ignorant of the language. He also committed maleficence—he gave her a diagnosis without having established 100 percent evidence of colon cancer cells.

Some two years earlier, Mama started asking me "Could it be that I have cancer? Look at this ball that I have here." She touched the upper right part of her abdomen. "Could it be that I have cancer in the liver? Touch me, look, touch me." I palpated her, but I did it as a daughter would do it, not as a doctor. I palpated her superficially, since Mama did not let me palpate her deeply. She said it hurt. Perhaps, deep inside of me, I did not try to palpate her correctly, as it should be done. She was not my patient. She was *mi madre*. Now I recognize that I was afraid to feel a tumor.

I reasoned that if a tumor existed, if it was malignant, malignancy would signify the end of her life. I imagined that because of her age and character, Mama could not bear to know that she had cancer. I thought that. Thus, I palpated her so superficially that I felt no tumor. Consequently, I made up my mind that what she felt as a tumor was one of the two abdominal-wall hernias that she had already had for years, and now, because of her age, they were more protuberant and obvious. At times you don't see what you don't want to see. This is a risk of being a physician and a kinship-caregiver.

Additionally, she had had a history of diverticula, so I told her that the abdominal pain might be diverticulosis because she was careless with her diet, but deep down, I knew of the possibility of cancer. The augury was present. For me the augury is a more heartfelt and aesthetically pleasing way to interpret a prognosis. The augury validates intuition, something the prognosis cannot. The prognosis talks about the probability that an event may happen in the future, one that we say will happen because we read signs and symptoms, which only accommodates reason.

When I said "the augury always haunted us," I remembered that in her thirties Mama was always constipated. She used to say that she "shit like a goat," in round balls, while in recent years the constipation was combined with frequent episodes of irritable bowel syndrome. However, chronic constipation is also a risk factor for developing colon cancer (American College of Gastroenterology 2012; Guérin et al. 2014).

The first strong suspicion I had that Mama had cancer arose when I came home after a month of travel for work. When I returned, it frightened me to see that Mama had lost a lot of weight—thirteen pounds in one month—despite eating as normal. She felt weak, fatigued, and more constipated than ever. Blood in the stool was visible to the naked eye. As we doctors say, Mama was "a textbook case"; that is to say, the patient met all the criteria described in the literature. Perhaps being informed of all these symptoms led the ER doctor to pronounce the diagnosis of colon cancer summarily while forgoing the indispensable results of a biopsy.

The rapidity with which we advanced through the system of medical referrals prompted me to forgive the ER doctor's hasty maleficence. At times, you must be practical and focus on the priority; in this case, the priority was to streamline the referral system with the gastroenterologist. We achieved that. We left the emergency room informed that we would receive a date for colonoscopy. I spent twenty-four hours a day with Mama. I supervised her diet, I was strict with every morsel of food she put in her mouth, and she was disciplined enough to reduce the inflamed colon before the colonoscopy was scheduled. It was critical to reduce inflammation to reach the tumor site to get the biopsy.

During the two weeks prior to the biopsy, Mama cooperated with her own care. She obeyed my every instruction. I was relieved, since this is unusual behavior for her. She generally ignores my recommendations, especially those to eat more fiber, drink more water, and decrease sugar intake. In a matter of weeks, I felt that the parent/child role was reversed (Williams et al. 2014); the negotiation to change roles was rather easy. Mama seemed as if she were a helpless girl putting herself in my hands, trusting my criteria as her only possible support. I was pleased that she facilitated the negotiation of our new behaviors but saddened to see such a strong-willed woman now fragile and dependent on me. I was not ready to become *mi madre's mama* (Simpson 2010). I did not want it.

I took care of shopping, making sure to include foods in her diet to prepare her as well as possible for surgery, but first for the colonoscopy. Considering her nutritional needs, I organized a diet alternating liquid and semiliquid recipes. Acquiring food to meet all the nutritional requirements with minimum sacrifice in taste greatly damaged our finances—but her well-being was well worth it.

A difficult task at this stage came after chemotherapy—preparing food for my ailing mama. Since I was a teenager, I had cooked only for myself. When I lived with Mama, she was "chief of the kitchen." I had never cooked for her before. In my adult life, my cooking style became very international; Mama does not completely enjoy my taste. Besides, since I react with a migraine to a wide variety of foods, I am very finicky about ingredients. Therefore, to stay well I eat the same thing for weeks, but Mama cannot stand monotony. She likes to vary our meals every day, even if she must prepare two different dishes—one for her, one for me. As for the strange things I made her eat, she joked that I almost poisoned her.

In addition to my difficulty in preparing adequate food for her and maintaining a pleasant taste, I was faced with inconvenience in using a kitchen and utensils not our own. If someone asks me what was the most difficult, apart from Mama's illness and treatment, it was living in someone else's house, losing the independence to which we were accustomed to in our own home, where there's no need to ask permission to do or to use anything.

Although I had difficulty satisfying Mama's palate, she was very kind and told me that everything was fine; she constantly thanked me for the effort I put into caring for her. That comforted me and calmed me down, since cooking was a way of expressing how much I cared for her and how much I loved her. Among Latinos/as, cooking for the sick individual is an expression of responsibility and love (Howe, Hinojosa, and Sheu 2019). Among Mexicans, we do this even among neighbors when they are ill.

Another difficulty I faced as Mama's caregiver was sharing a bed with her at my friend's house. The bedroom had only a single bed. I have slept alone all my life. Mama's every movement woke me up when she got up several times to go to the bathroom at night, and I had to accompany her to see if blood was in the stool. During her illness and treatment, she presented intermediate insomnia. I felt guilty for sleeping while she was awake, alone with her thoughts, thinking about her life and her fears.

During our nine months in California, I maintained full-time status as a professor at my university in Mexico, teaching three online courses. Facebook and email allowed me to maintain communication with my students. The university permitted me to work remotely even before the COVID-19 pandemic. I knew the starting date but no ending date. It was agony. Daily I lived with uncertainty, fearing that my supervisor would call me to return to teach face to face. Fortunately, that did not happen—it was an immense relief. Losing my remote position would have taken away what little joy I had. Without work as a distraction from caregiving, I would have become impatient and frustrated. Taking time for yourself is vital to reduce the overwhelming demands of constant caregiving. Distraction differs for individuals—television, yoga, dancing, conversation, support groups, or any hobby. For me, it was work.

Despite new caregiving responsibilities, I had to present myself and deliver lectures via video to teach classes remotely. I put on makeup. I dressed up, pretending I was energetic, happy, and carefree. The reality was that daily contact with students recharged me as I spent twenty-four anxious hours a day caring for and worrying about Mama. Despite pain, we kept each other in good company; in bad times, we did our best to strengthen each other.

The day of the colonoscopy arrived. I felt satisfied because the dietary management I had implemented with Mother had good results—they managed to do the biopsy. It was positive. It showed the presence of colon cancer. This seventy-eight-year-old woman who I thought would crumble at the definitive news of cancer remained stoic and brave. "I'm old, but I do not want to die yet. If you are going to take me away, God, I ask only that you not let me suffer. I have already suffered so much in this life. Do not let me suffer more." This is what Mamita told me she asked of God every day since the diagnosis of cancer. Mama wanted to live. She was willing to go through anything to stay alive.

When I heard Mama begging God like this, I felt helpless. It was beyond my power to prevent suffering from disease and treatment—just as it was beyond my power to prevent suffering from her past. As a daughter, and now caregiver, I could offer to accompany her, to be her cook, her nurse, her secretary, and her shoulder to cry on, and above all, to be the daughter who loved her unconditionally, who would never leave her alone in her illness—but I could never guarantee her a painless journey.

There followed days of many exams preparing for surgery. The MRI scan and PET scan were among the most complex and effective procedures to complete the colon cancer diagnostic. I found public transportation to reach the place for the PET scan in Sacramento. Over time, I became an expert in finding various offices and diagnostic centers by public transport. We had no car. We couldn't pay for Uber. I couldn't abuse my friend's kindness by borrowing her car. As a caregiver I had to be aware of all these contingencies and at the same time consider those who helped us.

Some weeks later, Mama was assigned the best surgical oncologist in Sacramento. I knew this because my role as a caregiver and daughter was to do research for Mama's tranquility, to guarantee she would be in the best hands. I googled him. He seemed to be about Mama's age. From the first day we met, we got along well with him. He was a simple, kind, fraternal person from the countryside, like Mama. He had worked picking tomatoes, peaches, and almonds. That, too, he had in common with Mama. At some point in life, each had been a fieldworker. The reviews of his work were all excellent. I felt Mama was in the best hands possible.

A few hours before the surgery, I spoke with Mamita, telling her that my brother and I had a request. "We want you to promise that if everything goes well in the surgery, you will leave the memory of our father in peace. You will never speak of him anymore. If you cannot forgive him, it's okay. Do not forgive him. But do not allow the memory of everything bad to keep destroying you." I told her between tears, "The damage our father did to you, all the stress he brought into your life, contributes to the cancer. Do not let it continue to damage your body."

Once again, I explained that stress, anxiety, and depression (Lillberg et al. 2003; Spiegel and Giese-Davis 2003; Soung and Kim 2015) contribute to the growth of cancer cells, progression, and metastasis. Mama promised to listen to us. The stressful, negative memory of our father's actions and words would never again be a reason for our conversations. We would only talk about him when there was something good to say. She promised.

At the time of the surgery, I felt fear and distress. I was afraid something would complicate the surgical procedure. However, what I feared most was that if Dr. Graves found metastases, he would say that he did not remove the tumor because the metastases were so extensive there was no point in removing it. If that were the case, it would only remain to give Mama palliative care and wait for death. All this drama and tragedy flashed through my mind. I thought that if this was her case, Mama would suffer terribly. It was what she asked God to prevent.

Furthermore, at that time, I failed to see myself as her caregiver. I had no idea that unconsciously I had adopted that role. I thought of myself only as a daughter who would never abandon her own mother in her hour of most need. What would it mean for me to care for a terminally ill patient? That did not cross my mind. In those moments, the caregivers annul themselves and think only about the life of the one who is sick.

On the day of surgery, our friend arrived from Salinas to stay with me in the waiting room. Fortunately, the company of our friend distracted me from my interior monologues. We entertained ourselves with funny dialogues, making me forget we were in the waiting room, waiting for news about Mama. My gratitude to my friend is immense to this day; the hours of waiting would have been dreadful without her by my side. Our friend loves my mother as her own because her mother died when she was a child. In my mother she found a loving person who has taken care of and worried about her since they first met. Such a female sorority offers comfort in times of crisis, when the world is too heavy to carry alone.

The surgery was quick and successful. Mama was out of danger. Dr. Graves performed a hemicolectomy, a surgical procedure by which he removed portions from the cecum to the first third of the transverse colon and part of the terminal ileum. Given the type and degree of cancer, he performed an omentectomy, removing all or part of the omentum with its fatty tissue, veins, arteries, and lymphatics.

The postsurgical diagnosis was colon carcinoma. Following the American Joint Committee on Cancer staging (American Cancer Society 2022), the colon cancer was diagnosed at stage 3A of five stages. It had spread to more than one nearby lymph node but not into the nodes themselves. Actually, from twenty lymph nodes removed and analyzed after surgery, only four were positive for cancer. At last, we'd received a good omen. Mamita had no metastases. Perhaps she was completely free of cancer cells.

A few weeks later, the postsurgical diagnosis was followed by a PET/CT scan of the skull base to midthigh, consisting of radioactive sugar (fluorodeoxyglucose) introduced into the blood. Cells that grow quickly are more likely to take up larger amounts of sugar than normal cells do. The body may show cells with areas of radioactivity in the PET/CT scan. If a patient shows no areas of radioactivity, doctors consider the patient a survivor free of cancer.

We waited ten days for the results of the PET/CT scan. The wait was agonizing for all of us. Based on the results, the oncologist might recommend chemotherapy, radiation, both, or none. If the PET/CT scan showed areas of radioactivity and the oncologist recommended chemotherapy, the treatment would be very aggressive and completely degrade my mother's body. Just as there are loves that kill, there are chemotherapies that kill too. Moreover, Mama was determined to stay alive.

Our dream was that no more treatment would be required, indicating we could go back to Mexico very soon to resume our daily lives without being a burden to others.

The cost of rent in Davis and its surroundings was inaccessible to us, making us depend on the hospitality of friends. The ten-day wait seemed eternal—more eternal than waiting for the biopsy that confirmed the diagnosis of cancer. Meanwhile, I continued my routine of cooking, caring for Mama's postsurgical wound, teaching classes online, planning consultations, and writing abstracts for a conference. Mama and I watched soap operas and movies on the tiny iPad to entertain and distract her in convalescence.

We saw the oncologist for results of the PET/CT scan; while waiting, I checked results of the exams on the electronic medical file accessed from the internet. Although I reviewed it every day, no results appeared. Perhaps it was a private data file only for the oncologist to see. One minute before the oncologist appeared, the results of the PET/CT scan showed up on my cell phone. "Impression: No compelling evidence for FDG (fluorodeoxyglucose) avid metastatic colon carcinoma is seen."

"Mama!" Elated, I exclaimed, "They found no more evidence of cancer!" Mamita's beautiful blue eyes and face brightened with joy. She could say nothing. At that moment, the oncologist—a very kind and gracious woman—appeared. Without preamble, she cheerfully said, "Victoria, I congratulate you! You are a survivor! We do not find more cancer cells in your body."

However, the doctor told us that Mama's stage 3 colon cancer required a six-month treatment of chemotherapy with infusion every two weeks to give her a 75 percent chance of destroying all cancer cells, or any nonavid fluorodeoxyglucose undetectable by PET/CT scan. Mama had the option to have chemotherapy or to risk that some cells not identified in the PET/CT scan could grow back, if they existed. Mama declared, "I want to stay alive as long as possible because I still feel useful. If chemotherapy helps me to live, I accept it."

In the ensuing months of chemotherapy, Mama's life was consumed by nausea; abdominal pains; diarrhea; burning sensations when defecating; depression; insomnia; anger; headaches; neuropathies in her hands, legs, and feet; mandibular tremor; anxiety; mouth sores; anemia; and—worst of all—loss of her sense of taste. For some months she could not appreciate the taste of food: "It's as if I am chewing cardboard."

During those agonizing months, we lived in an apartment where we felt more comfortable, thanks to a former student's cheap sublease. There we had privacy and freedom to reveal our tiredness, to cook, and to wander around the house during nights of insomnia and diarrhea.

More difficult days ensued as secondary effects of chemotherapy consumed Mama. She lost a lot of weight. Food no longer tasted good, its texture bland. To encourage her to eat, I bought miniature plates and glasses exclusively for her. Tiny portions garnered her acceptance. Without sense of taste and smell, once again Mama was kitchen commander in chief. She prepared meals, while I guided her on what and how much she should eat to avoid becoming malnourished despite losing weight.

Other patients arrived and stayed alone to receive infusions. I watched over Mamita by her side during twelve sessions of chemotherapy. She was the only patient in the chemotherapy infusion center with a companion. She fell asleep during chemotherapy while I read or evaluated my students' homework. The days of the month she felt strongest were infusion day and the day after chemotherapy. Every two weeks, after we left the infusion center, we went to Burlington to buy new clothes as her weight dropped drastically. Her clothes no longer fit.

Mom looked cute—new clothes, less weight, no alopecia, hair intact. I joked that she was the most fashionable patient at the infusion center: "See, Mama, patients are advised to dress in sportswear or loose clothing—but you look as if you walking on the red carpet." That spoke to her strong spirit. After a few weeks as kinship-caregiver, I got to know all the staff at the center. One week I traveled as a consultant to work in Guatemala and brought gifts for all the staff. We must show appreciation for staff and others caring for our loved ones.

Although Mama failed to keep her promise to bury the memory of our father, I began to understand that children have little right to ask parents to contain their emotions. Mama should feel free to think about whatever and whenever she wants. Besides, speaking about my father may be part of the healing process.

Six months later, Mama completed the recommended chemotherapy cycles. She remained strong, although chemotherapy damaged her peripheral nerves, resulting in neuropathy. She lost feeling in her hands, legs, and feet, causing difficulty with balance, and no longer felt safe when walking unaccompanied. Now she uses a cane to walk; if I offer my arm to lean on, she feels much safer moving ahead.

Now we live together. We are almost inseparable. Mama is eighty-two. Still she takes charge of cooking. I remain acutely aware of her medications, medical examinations, appointments, and rehabilitation while neglecting neither my work nor what I enjoy doing most—traveling. Even during the two-year blackout of the pandemic, sharing space with Mamita provided me the best company I could ever have.

Caregiving involves specific tasks that can be quantified and priced economically. I call them technical tasks. Such services are those that hired help can perform, but they also require other activities that Cristina Morini (2014) identifies as "untranslatable," and I add the qualifier "invaluable," because they lend such high value that it is impossible to calculate. Caregiving that you offer to loved ones implies emotional work, as Herminia Gonzálvez (2018) observes: rather than producing an object as a result, it produces life and well-being. This is invaluable. Gonzálvez (2018, 200) defines care work as "any activity—direct or indirect—that enables the multidimensional well-being of people, facilitating the development and maintenance of daily life."

When I started this journey of "caregiving" to and for Mama, I never imagined what it entailed. A leading economist of feminism, Amaia Pérez Orozco (2014), classifies caregiving tasks on three levels that require specialization: (1) to arrange material preconditions, (2) to deliver direct care activities, and (3) to dispense mental management activities.

Reading Pérez Orozco's work allowed me to write a checklist of tasks I performed as a kinship-caregiver and to realize that of the tasks Mama required, I performed them all. I confirmed that the tasks that best comfort a person you care for are those involving companionship, understanding, compassion, respect, teasing, joking, and affection—these tasks are the most difficult to provide. Those "untranslatable" and invaluable elements of caregiving represent values connecting us to an interdependent web of survival.

Caregiving implies activities involving the physical body and human emotions to satisfy basic organic needs of an individual who is ill. Caregiving entails feeding, giving medicine, monitoring diet, dressing, and bathing—direct care activities, or corporeal care. These needs are always present in the patient as part of the human life cycle. Such needs must never be neglected; the survival of the patient depends upon them: to pick up medications at the pharmacy, to do household chores that favor material preconditions, and to promote a person's well-being. The caregiver should try to elevate an ailing person's moods—putting household items in order, sanitizing living spaces, and beautifying the atmosphere and surroundings.

Caring for a sick family member demands much more specialized supervision, such as planning, controlling, and evaluating the process and progress (mental management activities) of the dependent person.

The list is long. The caregiver must initiate medical appointments, ascertain that appointments do not overlap, ensure that patients follow all instructions to prepare for examinations, administer care required for future procedures, monitor examinations, oversee results, accompany family members to medical consultations, explain to physicians important details omitted by patients, learn to interpret medical nomenclature, become aware of any change and urgent need, and, in many cases, arrange for necessary transportation and rehabilitation. Such intensive, critical caretaking may be routine in many hospitals, but it is not usual in family caregivers—despite the caregiver's love for an ailing dependent.

Accomplishing everything that caregiving demands and implies requires exceeding skill, ability, and emotional intelligence. These are traditionally assumed to be innate virtues of women—but they are not. We may also believe that the talents demonstrated by certain artists, writers, athletes, actors, or singers are innate. However, as professionals they are appreciated and paid for their endowment, while the laborious, stressful caregiving that women carry out is underestimated, uncapitalized (unpaid or underpaid), devalued, unnoticed, and often unseen.

María de los Ángeles Durán (2010) asserts that women—and, I believe, particularly those women who care for chronic or terminal illness—who overlap domestic work and provide caregiving, if they do all these at the same time in the same space with the same level of demand and the same injustice, could represent a ticking time bomb for themselves and for society.

Therefore, it is urgent to reeducate society so that everyone understands that caring for sick and nonsick relatives does not involve work expressed in the genetic makeup—as a natural attribute—of women, even though history presents women as essential caregiver subjects (Segato 2014).

Caring for family members must be recognized as a voluntary and supportive attribute essential for the survival of the human species and the planet (Arendt 2003; Nussbaum 2006; Carrasco 2017). If the legal and economic environment guaranteed justice, respect, appreciation, and compensation, then taking care of each other would be equitable, distributing the burden among family members. In this regard, Amaia Pérez (2006, 14) eloquently avows "that people are not autonomous or dependent, but that we are placed in different positions in a continuum of interdependence." Therefore, leaving caregiving exclusively in the hands of women inflicts an undue burden upon us, but it could also give us power that we could selectively stop exercising.

Taking care of Mama made me realize that autonomy confronted by illness is a mortal fallacy. Caring for Mama taught me the reality of interdependence, solidarity, and humility to understand that without support of others, when the moment of our own dependency arises, all of us need devoted caregivers by our side—or we may not survive.

Thank you tremendously for that, too, Mama.

References

American Cancer Society. 2022. "Cancer Staging." Last modified February 18, 2022, accessed January 23, 2008. https://www.cancer.org/treatment/understanding-your-diagnosis/staging.html.

American College of Gastroenterology. 2012. "Chronic Constipation Linked to Increased Risk of Colorectal Cancer." Science Daily, October 22, 2012. https://www.sciencedaily.com/releases/2012/10/121022081228.htm.

Arendt, Hannah. 2003. *La condición humana*. Buenos Aires: Paidós.

Beauchamp, T. L., and J. F. Childress. 1994. *Principles of Biomedical Ethics*. New York: Oxford University Press.

Carrasco, C. 2017. La economía feminista: Un recorrido a través del concepto de reproducción. *Ekonomiaz: Revista Vasca de Economía*, no. 91, 52–77.

DeVita, V., T. Lawrence, and A. Rosenberg. 2016. *Colon and Other Gastrointestinal Cancers*. Wolters Kluwer.

Durán, María de los Ángeles. 2010. *Tiempo de vida y tiempo de trabajo*. Bilbão: Fundación BBVA.

Englander, K., C. Yanez, and X. Barney. 2012. "Doing Science Within a Culture of Machismo and Marianismo." *Journal of International Women's Studies* 13 (3): 65–85.

Fallowfield, L. J., V. A. Jenkins, and H. A. Beveridge. 2002. "Truth May Hurt but Deceit Hurts More: Communication in Palliative Care." *Palliative Medicine* 16 (4): 297–303.

Flores, Y. G., L. Hinton, J. C. Barker, C. E. Franz, and A. Velasquez. 2009. "Beyond Familism: A Case Study of the Ethics of Care of a Latina Caregiver of an Elderly Parent with Dementia." *Health Care for Women International* 30 (12): 1055–72.

Gonzálvez, Herminia. 2018. "Género, cuidados y vejez: Mujeres 'en el medio' del trabajo remunerado y del trabajo de cuidado en Santiago de Chile." *Prisma social—revista de ciencias sociales*, no. 21, 194–218.

Guérin, A., R. Mody, B. Fok, K. L. Lasch, Z. Zhou, E. Q. Wu, W. Zhou, and N. J. Talley. 2014. "Risk of Developing Colorectal Cancer and Benign Colorectal Neoplasm in Patients with Chronic Constipation." *Alimentary Pharmacology and Therapeutics* 40 (1): 83–92.

Hallenbeck, J., and R. A. Arnold. 2007. "Request for Non-disclosure: Don't Tell Mother." *Journal of Clinical Oncology* 25 (31): 5030–34.

Howe, T. H., J. Hinojosa, and C. F. Sheu. 2019. "Latino-American Mothers' Perspectives on Feeding Their Young Children: A Qualitative Study." *American Journal of Occupational Therapy* 73 (3): 7303205110p1–7303205110p11.

Jensen, U. S., and G. Mooney. 1990. "Changing Values: Autonomy and Paternalism in Medicine and Health Care." In *Changing Values in Medicine and Health Care Decision-Making*, edited by U. S. Jensen and G. Mooney, 1–15. Chichester, U.K.: John Wiley and Sons.

Jotkowitz, A., S. Glick, and B. Gesundheit. 2006. "Truth-Telling in a Culturally Diverse World." *Cancer Investigation* 24 (8): 786–89.

Katz, J. 1986. *The Silent World of Doctor and Patient*. New York: Free Press.

Lillberg, K., P. K. Verkasalo, J. Kaprio, L. Teppo, H. Helenius, and M. Koskenvuo. 2003. "Stressful Life Events and Risk of Breast Cancer in 10,808 Women: A Cohort Study." *American Journal of Epidemiology* 157 (5): 415–23.

McCabe, M. S., W. A. Wood, and R. M. Goldberg. 2010. "When the Family Requests Withholding the Diagnosis: Who Owns the Truth?" *Journal of Oncology Practice* 6 (2): 94–96. https://doi.org/10.1200/JOP.091086.

Mendez-Luck, C. A., and K. P. Anthony. 2016. "Marianismo and Caregiving Role Beliefs Among U.S.-Born and Immigrant Mexican Women." *Journals of Gerontology: Social Sciences* 71 (5): 926–35.

Morini, Cristina. 2014. *Por amor o a la fuerza: Feminización del trabajo y biopolítica del cuerpo*. Madrid: Traficantes de sueños.

Nussbaum, M. 2006. "Poverty and Human Functioning: Capabilities as Fundamental Entitlements." In *Poverty and Inequality*, edited by D. B. Grusky and R. Kanbur, 47–75. Stanford, Calif.: Stanford University Press.

Pérez, Amaia. 2006. "Amenaza tormenta: la crisis de los cuidados y la reorganización del sistema económico." *Revista de economía crítica* 5, 7–37.

Pérez Orozco, Amaia. 2014. *Subversión feminista de la economía. Aportes para un debate sobre el conflicto capital-vida*. Madrid: Traficantes de sueños.

Segato, R. L. 2014. *La guerra contra las mujeres*. Madrid: Traficantes de sueños.

Simpson, C. 2010. "Case Studies of Hispanic Caregivers of Persons with Dementia: Reconciliation of Self." *Journal of Transcultural Nursing* 21 (2): 167–74.

Soung, N. K., and B. Y. Kim. 2015. "Psychological Stress and Cancer." *Journal of Analytical Science and Technology* 6 (30): 1–6.

Spiegel, D., and J. Giese-Davis. 2003. "Depression and Cancer: Mechanisms and Disease Progression." *Biological Psychiatry* 54 (3): 269–82.

Williams, K. C., E. M. Hicks, N. Chang, S. E. Connor, and S. L. Maliski. 2014. "Purposeful Normalization When Caring for Husbands Recovering from Prostate Cancer." *Qualitative Health Research* 24 (3): 306–16.

Zambrana, R. E., ed. 1995. *Understanding Latino Families: Scholarship, Policy, and Practice*. Thousand Oaks, Calif.: SAGE.

CHAPTER 8

The Reluctant Caregiver

The Complex Tale of Caring for My Mother-in-Law

MARIA ANGELINA SOLDATENKO

Maria Angelina Soldatenko's essay provides a nuanced vision of the caregiver: her story is that of the reluctant caregiver. This narrative is formed around the relationship between mother-in-law and daughter-in-law, although the broader contextual frame is familial. In contrast with familist renditions, the daughter-in-law does not embrace stereotypes of the Mexican woman *sufrida*. Her caregiver journey is marked by commitment and a need to engage in self-care, development, and self-preservation. She seeks a broader network of caregivers and an alternative educational path. Finally she points the reader toward a hard-wrought internal reconciliation with *la abuela*.

In this brief recollection of how I had to care for my mother-in-law when she got older, I try to come to terms with our past conflictual experiences and our reconciliation. First, I will honor her and recognize the strong presence and character of Abuelita Angelina, as we all called her. Abuelita cried every time she told us the story of her childhood and her sister, which I will retell below.

Abuelita Angelina

Abuelita was born in 1914 and came to live in L.A. in 1948 after living in Mexico City. Abuelita Angelina was raised at an orphanage by nuns with her older sister. Juanita, her sister, died of TB. Angelina left the orphanage at sixteen years of age. She was always hard working, organized, thrifty, and smart. She worked in sewing factories in California.

In the early 1950s, Abuelita met Gregory Soldatenko, a young Ukrainian man, at Evans, a school for English as a foreign language in downtown L.A. Gregory worked at a gas station. Their son, Michael, was born in 1953. Mike was twelve when their parents divorced in 1965. Abuelita became a single mother, kept the house, and continued working in sewing factories and renting rooms. She knew how to survive on her own while raising a child. By the time Mike was a teenager, Abuelita sent him on scholarship to a boarding school at a seminary. After graduating from high school, Mike attended Loyola University. By that time Abuelita had retired from work. She rented her home and attempted to live in Mexico. After a couple of years, she returned to Los Angeles because she could not adjust to life in Mexico. Mike and I got married in Mexico in 1972, against our parents' will.

Clash of Two Strong-Willed Women

Abuelita Angelina lived to be 104 years old and had dementia for many years. We are still grieving her loss. But also, we are at ease because she did not want to live bedridden, unable to do all the things that she loved. She was an amazing woman: hardworking, opinionated, and at times funny.

For me, it is important to reflect how I came to understand her, during her latest years in this world, and how I still did not totally understand how to deal with the fact that she suffered from dementia. I had to reconcile with the idea of embracing caregiving for the mother-in-law who for years had tried to make my and my husband Mike's lives miserable. By the time she became dependent on others, Abuelita was older and still fought us tooth and nail, as in the beginning. I had to engage in caregiving together with my husband because ethically that was our only option. I must explain that we were not on good terms with Abuelita, since I had dared to marry her son. I believed that I represented a challenge to her throughout. I confess that I did not help to make things better when I refused to practice Catholicism, pray the rosary with her, and attend Masses with her. Now I know that in part I reacted this way because I disagreed with the very conservative political positions of the church against women and gay people, but also because it was a means of defying her. I could probably have consented to join her, but she had been so wicked to me over the years that I could not stand her anymore.

And every time I stood up to her or dared to defy her in her most profound beliefs, I felt empowered.

I believe that Abuelita felt that I made the wrong choice in continuing my education. Her son could get an education. As a father, he could always aspire to that, but I, as a mother, should never attend university or pursue a graduate degree. Instead, I should only work and stay at home and serve Mike and the kids. According to Abuelita, it was wrong to hold intellectual interests after getting married to her son and giving birth. She was furious with every degree I worked for and earned. She never acknowledged my hard work, which would in the end benefit her son, her grandchildren, and eventually her as well. She missed this important connection. She was smart and independent, to have survived alone raising a child, but her dislike of me blinded her when it came to giving me any slack or final acceptance.

Abuelita wanted to break us apart, and to break us spiritually; she tried very hard. But the more pressure she used, the more united we became in our marriage and our family vows. She strengthened our bond with every attempt to keep us apart. For that I must thank her. She put us through fire. We came out victorious because we knew what we wanted and why we wanted it.

I did not become a caregiver to Abuelita out of choice; we did not have a strong bond. She was very close to her son, and she loved him, but she also seemed to live to make his life miserable. I learned how being the only child to a lonely, difficult mother can become a terrible burden to a son. She had planned to move to a Catholic retirement home in San Gabriel Valley; she would show us the brochure, which she kept. Ironically, she wanted to live her last years with nuns, mirroring her experience growing up in the orphanage. When Mike investigated retirement homes, he discovered that a decent one was very expensive. But even if we had been able to afford it, at the time, we could not have placed her in an institution like that; she was an integral part of our family. Mike would have been devastated. We decided to bring her home with us.

Legacy of Caregiving

I considered it our duty to take care of our elderly or sick, and I also cared for her out of compassion, because my husband, Mike, was her only son and she was my children's loving grandma. Also, Mike and I, as parents, had to teach our children about family duties. For me, it was also a chance to honor my mother's legacy of caregiving. My mother set the example as a caregiver for all our family in Mexico. My mother would have never forgiven me if Abuelita went to live in an institution. My mom cared for her elderly father with much love and attention.

My mom also prepared me to care and be of service. My mother was always sending her children on errands when anyone in our extended family needed us, when they got sick or needed help with babysitting. I still remember once, when I must have been maybe eleven years old, my mom left me at the Hospital General to spend the night with my grandma Trini after her eye surgery. I slept on the empty bed next to Granny. This is one of my earliest memories of caregiving.

I adored Grandma Trini. She was the most wonderful abuelita who told us stories and jokes and about how she survived the Mexican Revolution, hiding with her parents in the hills and dressing up as a boy to avoid being kidnapped or raped by men.

It became my destiny to care for Abuelita Angelina. It was expected of me to step up to the plate. I was not happy or at ease. She was very difficult to live with.

Caring as a Family for the Family: Illness, Religion, and Sisterhood

My sister Mago came to Pasadena from Mexico to be with me after my first surgery. Once in Pasadena, Mago loved to visit and pray the rosary with Abuelita or sit on the swing with her and talk. My sister would check up on Abuelita and keep her company. Both were devoted Catholics; they loved each other. That was when I found out that Abuelita had been prescribed a medication similar to one that my brother back in Mexico took. This particular medication was prescribed to bipolar patients. We were in shock, and we finally understood what was happening to her. For the first time we recognized that she was not well mentally. Her behavior and her demeanor were understood differently from then on. Nevertheless, it was still very hard to deal with her.

To take care of Abuelita, we needed a group of caregivers. The county provided a caregiver because Abuelita received both Medicare and Medicaid, since she never received much from Social Security. These assistants came and worked for twenty-five hours a week helping Abuelita. At that time,

Abuelita had mobility and energy. She went out with friends; some friends visited her, and some drove her to attend Mass.

Dementia: Not Recognizing the Symptoms

Abuelita used to call acquaintances and claim that she had been kidnapped by her family, taken against her will, abandoned to live in a terrible place. She told everyone who would listen that we were evil and that she was suffering. One of her old friends, Micaela, came once to check on Abuelita. She knocked and related to us how Abuelita had phoned her, crying that she was held against her will and begging her to save her and bring the police. Micaela came to check; she saw Abuelita's place and saw Abuelita in her garden.

Abuelita's calls also included calls to the police or fire department to report ill treatment. The firemen came often in the middle of the night. The paramedics would check her and find everything normal. They finally gave us an ultimatum: they would fine us if she raised another false alarm. We used to laugh and decry Abuelita's adventures. These stopped once we removed the phone line after some of these experiences.

It became clear to Mike and me that we would not survive working in academia, seeking promotions and tenure, and simultaneously caregiving for Abuelita. We lived with a lot of stress caring for Grandma with an illness that we had not identified timely and wisely.

Caregiving: Needing a Network of Dedicated Workers

Years later, when we went to live in Upland, things had changed, as Abuelita needed more help and constant supervision. We all lived in the same home; there was an area within the house for her. Again we all became a team. San Bernardino County limited the amount of time caregivers could provide to their client; in our case, it was twenty hours a week. These dedicated workers were a blessing to all of us; they were paid by San Bernardino County. Mike and I could not have survived caregiving without all of them. Both of us had to work as academics, an already stressful field of work to start, and by luck our sons were out of the house; we had sons in college or graduate school. Sometimes it was very difficult for us to negotiate caring for Abuelita.

My sons were never involved in caregiving. They did not have to live with her. Gabriel and Adrian were in college away from home for years, since the early 1990s, first completing their BA degrees. Adrian was in California at UCLA, and Gabriel at ASU in Tempe, Arizona, when Mike and I taught there. They both visited and enjoyed Abuelita's company. She was a different person with them; she loved her grandchildren and her great-grandchildren, who visited us every summer.

In time, we asked and privately hired my youngest sister, Lulu, who came to stay with us from Mexico, first for a few months; she ended up staying for almost four years. Lulu attended adult school to learn English during the day; then she would stay with Abuelita once the caregiver left. It was hard work for all of us; we needed to be efficient: cleaning after Abuelita, changing bedding, doing her laundry every day, bathing, and paying strict attention to her long list of medications and her diet. The most important aspect for all of us was to be very patient with her needs and demands. She was not terminally ill, just older. She had arthritis, high blood pressure, and high cholesterol, and now her mind was playing tricks on her. She needed help and understanding more than ever. She had concerns, but in general she was healthy and enjoyed a good appetite. She had never drunk or smoked when young; she had led a healthy life.

In Upland Abuelita needed attention twenty-four-seven. Abuelita would try to go out of the house and walk in the streets, although she needed a walker to move. We secured the front door with a series of locks. But even with all these precautions, she was able to open the front door one afternoon. Abuelita had been alone in her room taking a nap. She probably woke up, got confused, and went out the door! She tried to go down the steps with her walker. The neighbor across the street alerted us immediately. She fell down the front steps but fortunately suffered no injuries. When the neighbor tried to help, she screamed that he wanted to steal her walker! She kept us on our toes. We seemed to be stressed all the time. We could not leave her on her own, not even during her naps. After the first scare, the locks were also improved and harder to move. She was unable to leave or go out on the streets. The gates on the yard were secure as well. There was always someone near her most of the time when she could move a little. I was so attuned to her that at night I could hear her from upstairs. If she screamed for some reason, or if she had a bad dream, I woke Mike up. He went down to send her to sleep; sometimes she walked around in the dark.

Mike and I tried to have vacations as often as we could. For a while conferences became a way to get away. My sister Mago would come from Mexico; she would stay with Adrian and Abuelita back in those days. Mike and I discovered the beauty of distancing ourselves from both work and family obligations every summer. As soon as my grandkids could travel without their parents, we went away to Europe, only us four. Traveling with Mike and our grandchildren was, for me, the best medicine. We needed to go away to recover from the intensity of academic work combined with caregiving.

My sister Lulu stayed with Abuelita and became the primary caregiver when Mike and I traveled every summer. During our trip to Italy in 2017, my sister Lulu called us to come back, concerned by Abuelita's recent refusal to eat. Abuelita was becoming more frail. She slept most of the day and refused to eat or ate very little.

Abuelita had very little mobility. She was 104. We had set up a swing contraption to help her and to change sheets in her bed. She could no longer take a shower, even with the help of a chair and an assistant. Monica, the hired caregiver, gave her sponge baths and shampoos in bed. Abuelita mostly stayed in bed and slept. We were grateful that Abuelita had been healthy for many years. But now we were really worried about her. She prayed and sang every morning. She told us stories and made us laugh. She had a great appetite until she was 103, when we celebrated her birthday; she loved mangoes and guayabas. Abuelita was amazing; she read her books without glasses until she was in her midnineties. She was present and challenged us, arguing with Mike at any opportunity. She loved her independence. She outlived all her friends and family, but she still had a few younger friends that visited her, and she attended Masses until she became much older and opted for daily Masses on cable TV.

When my sister Lulu helped us, Mike and I were responsible for Abuelita's last diaper change at night, feeding her milk, and making sure she swallowed her night meds. Mike and I took turns at night. Mike and I were also responsible for any afternoon and evening accidents, often cleaning and changing her clothing and bedding—all needing to be washed. Once my sister Lulu returned to Mexico, it became harder for Mike and for me. We had to plan to help Abuelita before Monica, the caregiver, arrived every morning. Mike left at five thirty in the morning to park and catch the Metrolink to Cal State L.A. He could help only when he came back from work after five in the afternoon.

Mike had learned to change diapers, feed her dinner, and give her her night meds. If she woke up late at night, Mike had to go check on her.

Every morning before I went to teach at the college, just fifteen minutes away from home, I had just enough time to do my part. I got ready at five thirty in the morning. I walked the dogs at six o'clock. At seven or seven thirty, Abuelita would wake up, or I would gently ask her to awake. I brushed Abuelita's teeth, combed her hair, washed her hands, gave her a quick sponge bath if needed, and changed her diaper. Sometimes I had to also change bedding in the morning. Then I would prepare her warm milk and some bread, plus give her all her morning meds. I had to pay attention because now Abuelita had started to act out like a child, and she would refuse to open her mouth, or she would spit out her pills. I would not have a fit; I saw her as one of my children by this time. Before leaving for work around eight o'clock, I could observe how Abuelita was slowly slipping away. She would not even sit in her chair anymore. Her dementia now was more obvious. She would get anxious and ask me to bring her a bundle of fabric to sew because she had to make some money. She had been a garment worker in Los Angeles for many years to support her son. It was at these moments that she almost made me cry, and it dawned on me that she had been suffering from dementia for a long time. I tried to explain to her that she should not worry about money ever again, that Mike and I could cover any expenses. She would shake her head, dismissing me. She would laugh it off as if I were joking. I never contradicted her at that point. I'd read that we should just play along with dementia patients, not to confuse them more by trying to establish reality for them. I could never train Mike, who would try to reason with her, to make her understand. He would be upset that she was making up stories. Mike never recognized her dementia; he saw his mom as just having problems and driving him crazy by being contrarian. I know that it is hard for families to recognize dementia and mental illness among the people we are close to and love.

Abuelita passed in May 2018.

Conclusion

The process of reflecting about my reconciliation with Abuelita during her last years of living has helped me partially heal. Now, as a more mature woman, it has become clear to me that Abuelita suffered from dementia and that when I understood her behavior as an affront to me, this was my assessment as a young, immature daughter-in-law. Eventually, I came to see her actions as the result of her deteriorating health, which worsened with age. And I came to see that even if she felt, when she was still healthy, that I was not the best daughter-in-law, I should have accepted it and left it in the past. And by now I have learned to forgive her, and to forgive myself. It took me a long time to embrace and accept my role as a caregiver and as a daughter-in-law. This was the most difficult challenge that I had to face; ultimately, I had to accept Abuelita as she was. I feel that this experience of practicing everyday caregiving allowed me to become present, patient, and humble—in other words, a human being. The process of changing diapers, bathing, and dressing Abuelita was my atonement.

At the end of her days, at 104 years of age, she would wake up in the morning and say a prayer loudly: "*Gracias te doy gran Señor, porque con el alma en el cuerpo nos haz dejado amanecer, por tu caridad y amor nos dejes anochecer, en gracia y servicio tuyo y sin llegarte a ofender, amen*" (Thanks to thy Lord, because with our soul in the body you let us wake up. For your charity and love, let us be here tonight, in grace and service to you and without offending you, amen). That was my cue to go to her room. I would clean and change her, feed her warm milk and bread, and give her her meds every morning. However, when she overslept, I would get anxious. I would breathe in, I would say a silent prayer before going into her room, and I would approach her with fear of not finding her alive. Sometimes she would awake and smile.

I would try to express my sincere thoughts to Abuelita, who was no longer mad at me. I was trying to express this with my offerings of flowers in her room, with a small Christmas tree with lights twenty-four seven for months, and by authentically participating in caregiving. Finally, I was acting without resistance, without resentment, but feeling closer to her, trying hard to understand her. By then, I had learned to console her when she worried, without reason, about money and work. I tried hard to convince her that she was now surrounded by her family, who loved her, and by devoted caregivers. That all her hard work and devotion to her son had not been in vain. That all her suffering since childhood was now in the past.

I just hope that there will be caregiving roles for my sons, that it will not be as onerous for them as it was for us. When we took care of Abuelita with lots of help, we became sick. I went through two major surgeries and hospital stays. I just hope and pray that I will not live long enough to become a burden to my sons and family, and that I won't suffer from dementia or other terrible ailments. I wish I could just go to sleep and not wake up again. It torments me to think that my sons will have to be put to the test as we were.

I wish I could say that I foresee my sons taking on the caregiving role. They are good sons. I tried to teach them to resist patriarchy and the gender division of labor. They have learned to cook and clean after themselves. They observed from afar their parents dealing with caregiving Abuelita. They did not participate actively; they saw Abuelita only during some summer vacations and when they joined our family reunions to celebrate Abuelita's many birthdays. They did not benefit from learning about the tough experience of being a caregiver firsthand.

When we asked our sons what they would do if we become as old as Abuelita, if we need help and caregiving, if we become difficult, if we spit out our meds or have tantrums, one of my sons responded, in jest, that he would just put us both to sleep. The other son says that I should not worry about not been looked after. He says that it could never happen.

But Mike and I do not want or expect our sons to become our caregivers in the same manner that we became caregivers for Abuelita. We have planned for them not to feel that they must do it. We have prepared a fund so that they do not have to worry about us and expenses. But how can we ever be certain?

Among Latinas/os in the United States, it is expected that our elderly are not sent to retirement homes; we mistrust these institutions, as many have a questionable record. There is also the question of the affordability of a decent retirement home for our elders. Abuelita had a very low monthly Social Security check, which made her eligible for access to free medical care and equipment to make her comfortable, such as her wheelchair, bed, and swing to move her around the bed, as well as some hours a day of caregiving. Such care is not twenty-four seven, and many of the elderly need someone present around the clock. Thus, family members must come to the aid of their elderly, even with the assistance of paid caregivers, access to health care, and sometimes also disposable diapers. The state has transferred most of the caregiving work to families. Poor families pay the highest price with very few resources. The elderly who need caregiving but have no families suffer the most.

PART II
Community Caregiving

CHAPTER 9

Trauma and Caregiving

A Survivor and Caregiver Perspective

YVETTE G. FLORES

Yvette G. Flores's contribution presents readers a way to understand how caregiving takes different forms by providing an important illustration of how health care workers, in this case psychotherapists, can contribute to a fuller understanding of the administration of care within Latinx and Chicanx contexts. Her narrative surpasses contemporary doctors' narratives that focus primarily on their hidden stories; it demonstrates how interactions with patients can provoke meaningful transformations and critical insights. This piece also demonstrates the role that family and community members can play in assisting psychologists in healing unrecognized trauma. Finally, the essay identifies and highlights the importance of self-care and of the people and practices that support wellness and care in one's life, such as sisterhood with patients, women warriors, *comadres*, and *colegas*.

In this paper, caregiving is represented through a series of remembrances of exchanges and dialogues between my psychotherapy client, me in my role as therapist, and my own therapist. The piece highlights Latina mujerista (womanist[1]) decolonial practice, which in this caregiving process is embod-

1. Womanist and mujerista psychology centers values and worldviews that emphasize resiliency, strength, activism, self-expression, creativity, spirituality/connection, self-definition, and the struggle for liberation (Comas-Díaz 2020).

ied in the therapeutic and interpersonal relationships that take place between female caregivers and female care receivers who are united by trauma.

This essay challenges the orthodox and capitalistic modes of psychiatry and narrative health that are one-directional and distant. I write about how I was transformed by my caregiving and the exchanges with my client and, in turn, how my own therapeutic relationship binds us three women together, despite our different positionalities, age, class, and nativity. I, an immigrant Latina, and my psychotherapist, a Jewish woman whose grandmother was the sole survivor of genocide, share intergenerational and interpersonal trauma histories, which create nuance in our relationship and shape the *acompañamiento* I provide to my working-class Chicana emerging-adult client.

I argue that caregiving is multilayered and shaped by the caregiver and care receiver positionality; the relationship of caregiving is always evolving, and for it to be healing for all involved, it requires the therapist to be not only a vulnerable observer but an engaged, active participant in the healing process.

• • • •

We sit across from each other; she smiles, but the sadness in her eyes belies the apparent joy on her face. She is nineteen years old, a college student who heard me speak at a class in which I guest lectured on her campus and who would like to try therapy with me. There are no pressing issues, she states, other than that it is fall and she usually starts "strong," but by spring semester she has trouble completing her schoolwork and often has to leave school. She wants to make sure this doesn't happen again. We begin to discuss the usual rules of therapy: confidentiality, duty to warn, et cetera, et cetera, all the ethical requirements mandated by the state. She smiles. Within two weeks of therapy, she is in a fetal position under my desk, unable to speak. I ask her to draw what she is feeling. What emerges is a childhood and adolescence filled with violence and sexual abuse from her father and her brothers; her drawings are graphic depictions of physical, emotional, and spiritual violation (see Flores-Ortiz 1997). After the disclosure, she leaves my office, and I sit and cry.

I lie on my therapist's couch in the sacred space of her home office. I reached out to her years before, when I needed help negotiating a difficult separation from a mentor. I was her therapy client for fourteen years. She is Jewish American, a granddaughter of the Holocaust, an expert on state violence. She has traveled the Americas documenting the horrors of state violence in Chile, Nicaragua, Guatemala, and the United States. She knows that with a highly verbal and well-defended therapy client such as I, talk will get us nowhere. I can talk circles around most therapists. Therefore, she speaks, and I listen—I listen to my body, what it is telling me, what words cannot convey—while she guides. She monitors my breathing and asks what my body is telling me when she hears a change in my breathing pattern. She guides me to "my happy place." I was born on the Caribbean coast in Panama; thus, I assumed that my happy place would be the ocean. However, working with a Reiki master years before I discovered that my place of safety is a garden. It is filled with green foliage. It is sunny and warm. There is a sole bench along a path that leads somewhere, a place I have yet to visit. This is the bench where I sit when I need to feel safe and unviolated, where I can regain hope.

I lie on her coach and reenter my body. I can feel my skin, my bones, my mouth, my uterus, my vagina. The sites of so many violations for women. I invite the healing light to enter me and take away the pain, the shame, the tears that were not shed. My clients' pain, my mother's and grandmothers' pain, the ancestral shame and rage we carry as daughters of traumatized and violated women, we descendants of warriors and survivors.

This essay provides a *testimonio* of my caregiver work as a clinical psychologist for over thirty years. I examine the parallel process of giving and receiving care and the cultural assumptions that color my caregiving practices as well as the lives of my therapy clients.

Trauma and Healing

Guided imagery, hypnosis, meditation, artwork: these are some of the tools for recovery for survivors of state, social, family, intimate, and interpersonal violence. What happens when a person is violated, threatened, or assaulted or witnesses or directly experiences violence, whether it is verbal, emotional, physical, or sexual, depends on one's age, the frequency and severity of the abuse, and whether one receives any form of healing work. The younger one is, the more pervasive the impact of the trauma. My client was a small child when her father raped her. She was slightly older when her brothers began to sexually abuse her. The terror she experienced affected her neurobiology—her brain chemistry was altered.

When trauma, particularly physical and sexual violence, occurs in childhood, the child freezes because they cannot fight or defend themselves. Victimized children may manifest their distress behaviorally, in academic problems, pervasive sadness, *nervios* (Perry et al. 1995). In older persons, the fight-or-flight response is activated, but given the gender socialization around the world, women are more likely to freeze and cope through dissociation—the separation of mind/body/cognition/spirit. Over time, particularly if the abuse is frequent, the child or adolescent represses, or appears to forget, the violence that occurred. Dissociation and repression are ways to cope, to be able to go to school, to sit at the table next to the perpetrator and pretend everything is fine. My client can smile although she feels empty. Her smile is her mask. She needs to know she will be safe before she can show her pain, her wounds, her rage. Creating safety in the early phases of therapy is paramount for the client to gain the trust necessary to disclose the violence and to integrate mind/body/spirit in order to heal.

I can sit across from her and see through the façade because I, too, know how to dissociate. I, too, was a child when my cousins "played doctor" with me, when my uncle masturbated in front of me, when the family doctor (my uncle) examined me to determine why I had difficult menses and fondled me until I had an orgasm. I was a teenager when my boyfriend forced me to have sex with him. I did not know it was rape at the time because he claimed to love me and I was in love with his green eyes, his depression, and his *latinidad*. I used my dissociation to withstand the abuse of a Mexican lover and the unhappiness in my marriage. My closest male friend told me that I had a PhD in clinical psychology and a doctorate in dissociation. A male therapist once told me I did not have a brain, I had a top-of-the-line Pentium processor (this was in the 1990s); he wondered where I hid my heart.

My therapist can see through my *chingona* façade, my defensiveness, my intolerance of injustice, because she carries trauma in her own neurobiology. When one out of three women and girls in the world are victims of gender violence (WHO 2021), the likelihood of sitting across from a survivor is very high. As a clinical psychologist, I knew how to treat depression, anxiety, the wish to die. Those were the symptoms. When I first became a therapist in the early 1980s, no one talked about trauma, except in relation to veterans of war. We did not recognize to the extent we do today the battlefields of the home and the neighborhood, the injustice of the legal system, the maltreatment of women who dare report crimes committed against them. The multiple sources of female victimization and the risk factors now identified by the United Nations allow for an intersectional understanding, analysis, and treatment of gender violence (see United Nations 1979, UNODC 2009, and Bryant-Davis and Tummala-Narra 2018).

It is 1993. I have had my PhD in clinical psychology for eleven years. I have never had a course on the assessment, identification, or treatment of trauma. I had terrific training experiences with some of the best in the field. None of them, all men, ever discussed gender violence. I recall a difficult conversation I had in 1977, in supervision, when a Chicana female supervisor (the only one I ever had) told me that we could not do the group for abused women because the agency director, a Chicano, had told her that if we did, white people would use that as evidence that Chicanos and Mexicanos were in fact violent, abusive men. We had to keep the secret that our *familias* also rape and physically, emotionally, and verbally assault their members. We had to protect our male relatives, we were told, from the negative stereotype. Otherwise, he said, we would be considered (she and I) Malinches, traitors. We did not advertise it, but we ran the group. We called it a women's support group. The female staff began to refer to our group the women they knew who had been abused. Passive resistance, we called it in those days. Like my client, we smiled and pretended to follow the male director's instruction, masking our outrage in order to do what needed to be done. But we had had no training in the treatment of trauma. How were we supposed to do this? How were we supposed to help women heal from unspeakable offenses?

We had to remember who we were. We needed to reconnect to our ancestral knowledge. We needed to pray, do ceremonies, remember our traditions in order to heal. Mujerista psychologies (Gloria and Castellanos 2018; Comas-Díaz 2018) remind us that to heal from trauma means reintegrating, re-membering, body-mind-spirit (Flores-Ortiz 2001b). Before neuroscience pointed the way to how we can heal from intergenerational and current trauma, Indigenous and mestizo psychology (Duran and Duran 1997; Ramirez 1998) had shown us the way.

We know that trauma increases the risk of chronic illness later in life (see Enriqueta Valdez-Curiel's essay in chapter 10), as well as emotional, mental, and spiritual disorders, such as generalized anxiety disorder, panic disorder, and major depressive disorder. The *Diagnostic and Statistical Manual* of the

American Psychiatric Association, now in its fifth edition, defines trauma and provides criteria for the diagnosis. Posttraumatic stress disorder (PTSD) is defined as a serious psychiatric disorder that results from experiencing, witnessing, or hearing about a life-threatening event or events outside of normal experience, such as physical violence and threats of violence from family members. My client endured multiple experiences of terror and violence in her home. Her perpetrators were her father and brothers. The symptoms of PTSD often appear *after* a life-threatening event. While the violence is happening, many survivors describe leaving their bodies, floating away, observing what is going on without feeling it (Flores-Ortiz 1997). Given the multiple instances of violence, my client developed complex trauma. This is a more severe form of PTSD resulting from multiple exposures to life-threatening situations. When a child is not safe in her family, she cannot trust those who are supposed to protect her because they are the abusers; her fundamental sense of safety is destroyed.

There are four clusters of PTSD symptoms clients must have to meet the criteria for the disorder (see American Psychiatric Association 2022):

- Reexperiencing the event: spontaneous memories of the traumatic event, recurrent dreams related to it, flashbacks, or other intense or prolonged psychological distress.
- Heightened arousal: aggressive, reckless, or self-destructive behavior; sleep disturbances, hypervigilance; or related problems.
- Avoidance: distressing memories, thoughts, and feelings, as well as external reminders of the event.
- Negative thoughts and mood or feelings: blaming oneself or others for the traumatic event; feeling detached or disconnected from others; reduced interest in activities previously enjoyed; difficulty remembering important details of the traumatic event.

The survivor of the traumatic events also may feel guilty about the event(s); this includes experiencing survivor guilt. In addition, anxiety, stress, and tension are also common, and survivors may display the following symptoms:

- Agitation or excitability
- Dizziness
- Fainting

- Feeling one's heart beat in the chest
- Headaches

Trauma can affect every aspect of a person's life: how she relates to others; whether she can trust, laugh, make love; whether she feels entitled to parent, to be healthy, to enjoy life free from guilt and shame. Likewise, trauma has profound effects on memory. Many clinical studies of PTSD-diagnosed patients indicate that 70 percent of those patients experience dissociation (dissociative disorders) or "going blank," which explains the difficulties trauma survivors experience in recounting their histories of violence. The trauma is frequently reexperienced in the form of involuntary intrusive recollections, commonly referred to as flashbacks. In addition, the trauma is difficult to recall voluntarily; important parts may be totally or partially inaccessible—a feature known as dissociative amnesia. This was evident during Dr. Blassey Ford's testimony during Brett Kavanaugh's Supreme Court nomination hearings, when she had difficulty recalling the exact location of the party where Brett Kavanaugh assaulted her. In situations of stress, such as providing testimony, the traumatized individual may have trouble remembering important aspects of the trauma, become confused, or simply be unable to answer, as their nervous system is triggered by the hypothalamic-pituitary-adrenal axis and generates a fight-or-flight response, hyperarousal, and emotional dysregulation. In such cases, the individual may be experiencing dissociative amnesia. She simply cannot access the information voluntarily well enough to answer questions being posed to her. Survivors experience a dissociative continuum with intermittent fear and hyperalert responses that are not in their control (Wilde 2018).

Dissociation is viewed as a defensive or coping mechanism to prevent the trauma survivor from having to be overwhelmed by severely threatening images, memories, and flashbacks of past events, "People who have learned to cope with trauma by dissociating are vulnerable to continue to do so in response to minor stressors" (van der Kolk and Fisler 1995, 513), as well as significant stressors, such as recounting their history to a mental health professional or asylum officer or testifying in court. Studies also show a significant increase in posttraumatic intrusions—that is, higher prevalence and severity of trauma symptoms—and a significant decrease in posttraumatic avoidance and hyperarousal symptoms from before and after disclosing the abuse, and particularly when providing testimony in criminal or immigration proceedings or asylum interviews (Schock, Rosner, and Knævelsrud 2015). After testifying in court, traumatized individuals tend to experience greater severity of trauma symptoms and a reduced ability to avoid thinking about the traumatic events. This in turn increases anxiety and depression. The same can occur after a disclosure of abuse.

After an initial disclosure of abuse, therapy clients may flee from therapy, as the increase in symptoms may increase the guilt, shame, and pain of breaking the silence. Furthermore, a number of studies (including Dekel and Bonanno 2013; Staniloiu and Markowitsch 2014) suggest that repeated telling and interviews often alter the narratives of trauma survivors because of the increased symptomatology (hyperarousal, dissociation). A failure to understand these neurobiological processes can lead to false assumptions that the victim is lying or fabricating the abuse, or simply being "resistant" to or in therapy.

"How do you do it, Chula?" my Mexican male colleague asks. How do you sit day after day dealing with trauma, listening to these stories? How do you deal with this? I had run into his office after my client disclosed, through pictures, the extent of her abuse. He and I have been friends for years, since we met while we were both in graduate school. We started a private practice together; we often consulted with each other because we respected our gender perspectives and understood, despite our differences, that as Latinxs in the United States, at times we felt like fish out of water. We were part of a Latinx therapist network for years. "I don't know," I responded.

After each session with a trauma survivor, I drove home and looked at my children and inquired about their homework. I hugged and kissed them and hid my tears until I could not breathe. In other words, I dissociated. I turned the dial and pretended all was fine in the world. And I danced. I went back to dance classes and went to the gym regularly to work out. I also wondered, How does my colleague not deal with this level of trauma in his caseload? Does he not see it? Does he not feel it? Does he not recognize the victimization in his clients? Is he not hyperalert, on guard, seeing abuse everywhere, as my then husband claimed I did? He is a Mexican Jew; there is trauma in his genealogy, but have his class and male privilege protected him from seeing trauma in his therapy clients? And if he does, how does he deal with it? Does he also turn the dial? How do we provide care—become caregivers—in the face of such trauma? How do we negotiate the cultural rules that silence victims and protect the victimizers?

Caregiving and Receiving in the Context of Trauma

Traditional notions of caregiving situate women primarily as the providers of care within families. Daughters, wives, and daughters-in-law are expected culturally to raise children and to support spouses and elders within the families. As contributors to this volume poignantly articulate, culturally based forms of caregiving can create emotional burdens, lead to burnout, and contribute to physical illness. Little in the literature sheds light on Latina feminist notions of caregiving. How do we, as Latinxs, challenge traditional notions of *familismo* and derive more balanced notions of lovingly providing care? My earlier work on caregiving elders with dementing illnesses (Flores et al. 2009) called into question culturally rooted familistic notions of caregiving.

Likewise, my cultural upbringing created prohibitions against disclosure of intrafamilial abuse, which tacitly revictimize those victimized and facilitate abuse with impunity. I began to denounce, in my writings, the structural and cultural factors that propitiated and maintained gender violence in Latinx communities (Flores-Ortiz 2001c, 2003). At the time, however, I did not see my therapist role as that of a caregiver.

I was trained as a clinical psychologist with an ideology of clear boundaries between therapist and client. Ultimately, the therapy client is to be responsible for their own healing. As a Latina community clinical psychologist, I knew that my Latinx clients did not heal alone. They needed a supportive community to face and transcend the racial, sexual, and interpersonal traumas that affected their bodies/minds/spirits. I was part of that community. I was not an objective outsider providing tools the client could use to heal. My family therapy training from a humanistic intergenerational perspective suited my cultural values best. I was part of the system of care that facilitated healing. Supporting the healing from trauma of others required me to address and heal my own victimization and to better understand the intergenerational trauma transmitted in my family. Without my own healing, the risk of burnout was high.

What is the cost to the caregiver of clients with trauma? We now have a term for it: compassion fatigue, or secondary trauma. Back in the 1990s, I began to feel saturated by all the stories of abuse I was hearing from mostly women clients. A few men had heard that I was an ally to the Latinx LGBTQ communities and sought therapy with me. Others came because they knew about my politics, and others because they knew people who knew people who recommended me. At one point, I had twenty-five clients I saw weekly. They all were survivors of sexual violence. I also was teaching full time as an assistant professor. I had two school-age children and a failing marriage. I applied for a Fulbright Fellowship and went to Panama for a year. It was an elegant version of a trauma response. I fled. I transferred my clients to other colleagues who could address anxiety, depression, PTSD—trauma.

In Panama my plan was to teach and decompress. I did not plan to do any clinical work. I needed time to deal with my compassion fatigue. However, the Creator and the universe appeared to have other plans for me. One of the students in the family therapy class I was teaching approached me and invited me to meet with some of her colleagues; they had started a program through Caritas, a Catholic organization, to provide legal and counseling support to women in abusive relationships. It would only be an informal meeting, over coffee, she said. In that meeting I was introduced to the Panamanian regional director of the Network Against Violence Towards Women and Girls. She invited me to do a training based on my work experiences.

Within a few weeks, I was consulting weekly, doing trainings, and supervising. I also was dealing with my mother's family, who embodied the legacies of colonialism and U.S. intervention. I also arrived in Panama after the U.S. invasion of 1989. The country was traumatized. A sequela of that violence was an increase in child abuse and intimate partner violence in the general population. I had left the belly of the beast and arrived at one of its principal victims. I began to do co-therapy with a colleague from the university and offer consultation to the clients who used the university training clinic and my colleague's private practice. At the clinic we saw working-class families struggling with family injustice, economic disparities, and the losses of family members due to addiction and the U.S. invasion. In the private practice we saw affluent and middle-class Panamanians who were involved in custody battles and difficult divorces due to spousal abuse. Many of the women came in vehicles with armed bodyguards provided by their fathers to protect them from violent estranged spouses who had cartel connections. I pretended to be fine. I was terrified and constantly hyperalert. I did not tell anyone about the stories I was hearing.

I was invited to a press conference where subsequently I was demonized for talking about the incidence of violence in the country. I made front-page news in the country's main newspaper, *La Estrella de Panamá*. My mother's eldest son chastised me. How could I embarrass him by speaking out about men's violence? How could I associate with feminists and bring shame to his family name? He, the philanderer and emotionally abusive spouse whose wife took out her rage on her male children, had the audacity to try to silence me. He had become aroused when he danced with me when I was eighteen and he was thirty-eight years old. Now he was ordering me to be quiet. Instead, I accepted an invitation by the first lady of the Republic of Panama to speak to the wives of all the ministers at a breakfast. I began my talk by reading a poem written by my therapist. It was a poem about silence, about violence, about resiliency, about hope. All the women cried. The male journalists left the room. The event was not covered in the news.

I come from a long line of psychics, herbalists, and healers. I rejected the gift of "seeing" because I saw the toll it took on my mother to know things before they happened. She lived with anxiety and sadness. Some argue that trauma opens the psychic channels (see Valdez-Curiel 2001). From a neurobiological perspective, perhaps trauma and its resultant hyperarousal allows survivors to see beyond the conscious plane. At any rate, both my children have the *don*, the gift. One afternoon as I was getting ready to leave to go teach, my son pleaded with me not to go. I told him I had to. It was my responsibility; I had to go to work. He pleaded as I left. Shortly after I arrived on campus, I fell. Despite the pain, I proceeded with my lecture. One of my students insisted that I see the school nurse, who came to the classroom and wrapped my foot while I taught. After class, I could not walk: the pain was unbearable. One of the students insisted on driving me to the hospital. The dean met me there. She and my student were middle-class professional women. They had connections, given their social status. My student called her orthopedist at home and asked him to come to the hospital to see "an important professor from the U.S." who had fallen and was in pain. The doctor arrived quickly and, after x-rays, informed me that I would not be dancing at the next carnival. I had a broken foot. He ordered a cast and told me not to move for three weeks. I went back to teaching the next week.

I had not listened to my son, and I did not listen to my body's message or the physician's directive. I kept on doing everything I had *not* planned to come to Panama to do. My cast had to be replaced three times because it would break due to my walking on it. The doctor would shake his head and call me *terca* (stubborn). At the end of my stay in Panama, I returned to the United States with a lot more knowledge about the treatment of trauma, but it would be nearly twenty years before I would really listen to my body.

During this time, advances in neuroscience began to prove scientifically what our ancestors had taught us for millennia. Trauma causes *susto, espanto,* an *arrebato* (Anzaldúa 2002), a dismemberment. We become disembodied, disconnected from our physical selves in order not to feel the pain, the *agravios* (Flores-Ortiz 2001a). We repress, we forget, but the body remembers.

In 1998 I joined a group of Latinas who wanted to do collaborative research. Our meetings evolved into *Telling to Live: Latina Feminist Testimonios* (Latina Feminist Group 2001). While on retreat in the Sangre de Cristo Mountains, I began to dream and to write from the heart. I began to re-member my own experiences of victimization. I began to document my own healing journey (Deeb-Sossa et al. 2015; Flores-Ortiz 2001a, b, c, d; Flores-Ortiz 2003). I stopped silencing my own narrative because, after all, I had not suffered as much as others. But I remained a workaholic, largely because the academic path to success demands it. I began to lose friends, women my age and younger, who succumbed to cancer, brain aneurysms, accidents. I could not ignore the message from the Creator. I began to seek alternative healing strategies.

Once, while I was waiting for my massage therapist, a Native American / Italian American woman, her Native American mother walked by the waiting room and, hearing my difficulties breathing, stated, "Yvette, wouldn't it be easier to just cry?" To my surprise I could not tell her that in my family women do not cry. We were taught that crying was a sign of weakness. We are warriors. So, I had to learn to weep, to purge ancestral and personal wounds through tears so that I could breathe. I know my asthma is trauma related. It first manifested during the Anita Hill hearings. It came back with a fury during the Kavanaugh confirmation process. Another perpetrator wins. I told my body that it need not punish itself to express outrage. There are other ways.

I am a healer who needs healing. I carry the sorrow of others, and I am not able to let it go some of the time. I am now an elder. The agravios in my life are manifesting in my body with a fury. My knees began to hurt around 2016. There were days I could barely walk. I began to reflect on what was forcing me to be still, to lie down, to walk slowly, more carefully. I asked myself what it was I no longer wanted to do. While I was recovering from knee surgery, the COVID-19 pandemic arrived, forcing those of us with privilege to stop, shelter in place, and find alternative ways to work (if we had to). In my case, I had to learn to teach remotely, hold meetings via Zoom, and support my grandchildren and children emotionally as they negotiated the reality that came upon us.

How could we continue to provide care for those who depended on us—family, students, therapy clients, supervisees, immigration clients? I began to practice mindfulness, returned to yoga as a weekly practice, and opened my heart again to the possibility of love. I continued to practice my caregiving role as an individual and family therapist and psychological evaluator of clients in immigration proceedings, particularly asylum cases. My caregiver work was guided by the tenets of mujerista psychology (Bryant-Davis and Comas-Díaz 2016). This approach to therapy emphasizes the resiliency and strength of women of color that result from and manifest in activism, creativity, and self-expression. Moreover, mujerista psychology foregrounds the importance of self-definition and the connection to women's spirituality. Ultimately, the approach promotes the liberation of all who have been oppressed. These are values promoted by liberation psychology (Martin Baro 1994; Comas-Díaz and Torres-Rivera 2020), a psychological approach that aims to actively understand the psychology of oppressed and marginalized communities by conceptually and practically addressing the oppressive sociopolitical structure in which they exist.

These approaches to therapy are trauma informed and recognize that self-care is essential for balanced caregiving. Doña Enriqueta Contreras (2005), a Oaxacan elder *curandera*, told me years ago that *curanderas* stop healing others after age sixty or so because they need that energy to live. Instead, they continue their mentoring and training of apprentices and find other ways to promote community healing. This was an important message about self-care in the context of being a caregiver. Yet I continue to feel the burden of responsibility that accompanies my education and training. I still do too much. I feel too much. I am now embodied most of the time. However, I no longer need to dissociate in the presence of another's pain, as I have done a lot of healing of my own trauma. During the pandemic I was often triggered; thus I increased my mindfulness and yoga practice. I focused on my body.

In my conversation with my knees, they began to yell "STOP." I began to pay attention. I now have greater clarity. Yet there is still so much work left to do. I emailed my former therapist, who is semiretired. She tells me that stopping is overrated but slowing down is good. She always provides sage advice. This time I will listen.

References

American Psychiatric Association. 2022. *Diagnostic and Statistical Manual of Mental Disorders, Fifth Edition, Text Revision (DSM-5-TR)*. Arlington, Va.: American Psychiatric Association Publishing.

Anzaldúa, Gloria. 2002. "Now Let Us Shift . . . the Path of *Conocimiento* . . . Inner Work, Public Acts." In *This Bridge We Call Home: Radical Visions For Transformation*, edited by Gloria Anzaldúa and AnaLouise Keating, 540–79. New York: Routledge.

Berntsen, Dorthe, and David Rubin. 2014. "Involuntary Memories and Dissociative Amnesia: Assessing Key Assumptions in PTSD Research." *Clinical Psychological Science* 2 (2): 174–86.

Brönimann, Rebecca, Jane Herlihy, Julia Müller, and Ulrike Ehlert. 2013. "Do Testimonies of Traumatic Events Differ Depending on the Interviewer?" *European Journal of Psychology Applied to Legal Context* 5 (1): 97–121.

Bryant-Davis, Thema, and Lilian Comas-Diaz, eds. 2016. *Womanist and Mujerista Psychologies: Voices of Fire, Acts of Courage*. Washington, D.C.: APA Publications.

Bryant-Davis, Thema, and Pratyusha Tummala-Narra. 2018. "Cultural Oppression and Human Trafficking: Exploring the Role of Racism and Ethnic Bias." In *A Feminist Perspective on Human Trafficking of Women and Girls*, edited by Nancy M. Sidun and Deborah L. Hume, 146–63. New York: Routledge.

Comas-Díaz, Lillian. 2018. "Mujerista Psychospirituality." In *Womanist and Mujerista Psychologies: Voices of Fire, Acts of Courage*, edited by T. Bryant-Davis and L. Comas-Díaz, 149–70. Washington, D.C.: APA Publications.

Comas-Díaz, Lillian. 2020. "Journey to Psychology: A Mujerista Testimonio." *Women and Therapy* 43 (1–2): 157–69. https://doi.org/10.1080/02703149.2019.1684676.

Comas-Díaz, Lillian, and Edil Torres-Rivera. 2020. *Liberation Psychology: Theory, Method, Practice, and Social Justice*. Washington, D.C.: APA Publications.

Contreras, Enriqueta. 2005. "Traditional Mexican Midwifery: Doña Enriqueta Contreras." *Midwifery Today with International Midwife* 76 (Winter): 58–9, 69.

Deeb-Sossa, Natalia, Gloria M. Rodriguez, Ines Hernández-Ávila, and Yvette Flores. 2015. "CAR[T]AS: Rooting our Purpose as Academics in a Time of Transformation." In *El Mundo Zurdo 4: Selected Works from the 2013 Meeting of the Society for the Study of Gloria Anzaldúa*, edited by T. Jackie Cuevas, Larissa M. Mercado-Lopez, and Sonia Saldivar-Hull, 63–80. San Francisco: Aunt Lute Books.

Dekel, Sharon., and George Bonanno. 2013. "Changes in Trauma Memory and Patterns of Posttraumatic Stress." *Psychological Trauma: Theory, Research, Practice, and Policy* 5 (1): 26–34.

Duran, Eduardo, and Bonnie Duran. 1995. *Native American Postcolonial Psychology.* Albany: State University of New York Press.

Flores, Yvette, Ladson Hinton, Judith Baker, Carol Franz, and Alexandra Velasquez. 2009. "Beyond Familism: Ethics of Care of Latina Caregivers of Elderly Parents with Dementia." *Health Care for Women International* 30 (12): 1055–72.

Flores-Ortiz, Yvette. 1997. "Voices from the Couch: The Co-Construction of a Chicana Psychology." In *Living Chicana Theory,* edited by Carla Trujillo, 102–22. Berkeley: Third Woman Press.

Flores-Ortiz, Y. 2001a. "My Father's Hands." In *Telling to Live: Latina Feminist Testimonios,* edited by Latina Feminist Group, 33–38. Durham, North Carolina: Duke University Press.

Flores-Ortiz, Yvette. 2001b. "The Prize of the New Cadillac." In *Telling to Live: Latina Feminist Testimonios,* edited by Latina Feminist Group, 201–3. Durham, N.C.: Duke University Press.

Flores-Ortiz, Yvette. 2001c. "La tra(d)icion." In *Telling to Live: Latina Feminist Testimonios,* edited by Latina Feminist Group, 204–6. Durham, N.C.: Duke University Press.

Flores-Ortiz, Yvette. 2001d. "Desde el divan: Testimonios from the Couch." In *Telling to Live: Latina Feminist Testimonios,* edited by Latina Feminist Group, 294–97. Durham, N.C.: Duke University Press.

Flores-Ortiz, Yvette. 2003. "Re/membering the Body: Latina Testimonies of Social and Family Violence." In *Violence and the Body: Race, Gender, and the State,* edited by Arturo Aldama, 347–50. Bloomington: Indiana University Press.

Gloria, Alberta M., and Jeanett Castellanos. 2018. "Latinas poderosas: Shaping Mujerismo to Manifest Sacred Spaces for Healing and Transformation." In *Womanist and Mujerista Psychologies: Voices of Fire, Acts of Courage,* edited by T. Bryant-Davis and L. Comas-Díaz, 93–120. Washington, D.C.: APA Publications.

Latina Feminist Group. 2001. *Telling to Live: Latina Feminist Testimonios.* Durham, N.C.: Duke University Press.

Martin Baró, Ignacio 1994. *Writings for a Liberation Psychology.* Cambridge: Harvard University Press.

Perry, B. D., Ronnie A. Pollard, Toi. L. Blakley, William I. Baker, Domenico Vigilante. 1995. "Childhood Trauma, the Neurobiology of Adaptation, and 'Use-Dependent' Development of the Brain." *Infant Mental Health Journal* 16, no. 4 (Winter): 271–91.

Ramirez, Manuel. 1998. *Multicultural/Multiracial Psychology: Mestizo Perspectives on Personality and Mental Health.* Oxford, U.K.: Jason Aroson.

Schock, Katrin, Rita Rosner, and Christine Knævelsrud. 2015. "Impact of Asylum Interviews on the Mental Health of Traumatized Asylum Seekers." *European Journal of Psychotraumatology* 6, no. 10. https://doi.org/10.3402/ejpt.v6.26286.

Staniloiu, Angelica, and Hans J. Markowitsch. 2014. "Dissociative Amnesia." *Lancet Psychiatry* 1, no. 3 (August): 2236–41.

United Nations. 1979. "Convention on the Elimination of All Forms of Discrimination Against Women." See text at UN Women (retrieved February 24, 2022): https://www.un.org/womenwatch/daw/cedaw/text/econvention.htm.

UNODC (United Nations Office on Drugs and Crime). 2009. *Global Report on Trafficking in Persons*, February 2009. UNODC. http://www.unodc.org/documents/Global_Report_on_TIP.pdf.

Valdez-Curiel, Enriqueta. 2001. *Las curanderas de Zapotlán el Grande, Jalisco*. Guadalajara: Universidad de Guadalajara.

van der Kolk, Bessel A., and Richard Fisler. 1995. "Dissociation and the Fragmentary Nature of Traumatic Memories: Overview and Exploratory Study." *Journal of Trauma Stress* 8, no. 4 (October): 501–25.

WHO (World Health Organization). 2021. "Violence Against Women." World Health Organization. March 9, 2021. https://www.who.int/news-room/fact-sheets/detail/violence-against-women.

Wilde, Susan. 2018. "Precis on Trauma and Memory." Unpublished document to assist the evaluation of trauma survivors seeking immigration relief. Word document provided by the author, May 1, 2019.

CHAPTER 10

Caring for Students

An Act of Social Justice in Academia

MÓNICA TORREIRO-CASAL AND NATALIA DEEB-SOSSA

Mónica and Natalia's essay underscores the importance of understanding how caregiving takes different forms, including that of the interactions between instructors with their students. This essay highlights the impact that academia and caregiving for students has on Latinas in a predominantly white academic institution.

At a major public event at UC Davis, where we both teach, Angela Y. Davis gave a powerful speech titled "Social Justice in the Public University of California: Reflections and Strategies." To a full house, she challenged the UC Davis community to critically imagine a "feminist university." Davis asked, "How might we as students and faculty link our teaching, our research, our learning to . . . radical social transformation?" (2012).

We have always seen our work as faculty as radical/caring and as transformative. Our approach to our pedagogies mirrors the pedagogies of the home, by which *las familias* (families) equip their students to surmount their experiences at schools and other oppressive institutions that "often exclude and silence them" (Delgado Bernal 2001, 624). We also draw on feminist transborder thinking (Cervantes-Soon and Carrillo 2016) as we center students', their families', and communities' knowledges—critical awareness of borders crossings across geopolitical boundaries, institutions, languages, and ways of doing—to push against deficit messages of their educational promise (Dyrness 2011; Oliveira 2018). In our classes we honor the migration stories of our students and call attention to "our beauty, pride, and resilience in the face of inequality and injustice" (Favianna Rodriguez, quoted in Lee 2013).

Our caring pedagogy is founded in actively addressing the sense of isolation and marginalization students feel at UC Davis and actively creating a *sentido de pertenencia* (sense of belonging) by showing our *alianza* (social alliance), *solidaridad* (solidarity), and *apoyo* (support) to our students. It is at the Department of Chicana/o Studies and in other community settings that, together with our students, we have been able to create and find our *comunidad* (community) and a familia. It is *en familia* and in comunidad that we thrive, operate, and transform realities in an academic structure that prioritizes and rewards individualism and competition, as well as other patriarchal and divergent principles, rather than caring for others. In our understanding of our roles as educators, community members, activists, and mentors, caring for our students and their communities *is* part of our pedagogy. This caring pedagogy is not valued, as it is easily ignored in career promotions and discounted in academic settings.

During the pandemic, we faced very difficult times, and caring for our students was even more necessary. Most of our students are part of mixed-status families and have family members who are essential workers or are essential workers themselves. During the pandemic, our caring pedagogy implied a huge expenditure of our body-mind-spirit (Lara 2013), as we are actively listening to our students. We read their papers, and we support them to continue with their academic journeys. We know they represent hope for their families, who made sacrifices, left their countries of origin for better opportunities, and resisted racialized and gendered abuses.

We care for students struggling while we care for our own loved ones and worry about family members in other countries whom we cannot visit. We care despite the increasing toll our work takes, academically and personally. We care for our relatives at home while we work with the limitations of an online teaching system, which has forced us to change the interactive and personal nature of our classrooms. Despite the challenges, we continue to bring love, care, and creativity to our work. We spend hours writing letters of recommendation, providing guidance with applications, and helping students with their writing when our first language is not even English. We sit with them or with their families if necessary; we volunteer; we do community work; we advocate at school setting, in IEP meetings, and in diverse health settings.

Our Journeys to Academia: Becoming Feminist Scholars

As immigrant women coming from Spain and Colombia, respectively, we have encountered different militarized, settler colonialist, and capitalist academic institutions. As activist scholars we are constantly promoting and teaching curriculum that is antiracist, antisexist, and antihomophobic without seeing transformative structural change or healing from these forms of violence. We both feel disappointed, angered, frustrated, and *corajudas* (angry) when witnessing how the administrations—the university's and the U.S. government's—disregard our Chicanx and Latinx[1] students as merely a statistic, tokens, or a source of funding, dehumanizing their experiences and neglecting to acknowledge their concerns, demands, and dreams.

We are feminist instructors and activist scholars who have similar theoretical foundations and approaches in our work, teaching, social involvement, and interpersonal interactions with our students. We, as feminist scholars and political individuals, believe that to care for our students is an act of social justice. We share the urgency of working toward creating a feminist university which "cares" by actively transforming the lived realities of our students through a pedagogy that is inclusive, promotes changes, and involves students as proactive members and participants on campus and at community settings.

This pedagogy aligns with the Chicana/o movement principles of activism, engagement, and service to the community and the principles of a liberation pedagogy (Freire 1970). As immigrants, we also rely on and learn from our department mentors, such as Professor Chabram and Professor Flores. Their work as Chicanx activists and scholars is an inspiration and helps us to find balance and comfort during difficult times. We feel *arropadas* (protected) by their care and knowledge and the work that they have accomplished for all of us. As Flores (2015, 128) mentions, "Each of us is accountable to those upon whose shoulders we stood to get ahead. Those of us who have benefited from educational opportunities and have gained the privilege of an education can demonstrate that we did not stop being

1. We use, in attempts toward inclusivity and considering intersecting areas of privilege and oppression, the identifiers *Chicanx* and *Latinx* (pronounced *Chican-ex* and *Latin-ex*, respectively) as a way to move beyond the masculine-centric *Chicano* and the gender-inclusive but binary-embedded *Latina/o* or *Latin@*.

Latinx to get ahead. A commitment to social justice and spiritual activism is necessary for 21st-century scholarship." The solidarity, compassion, and caring for others and us often means a difficult balance, but as immigrant women we have brought hope and resilience to overcome challenges within our communities.

Although we grew up in different countries—Spain and Colombia—we have experienced similar *llagas* (wounds), through the deployment of dividing structures of power that have marked our bodies, nations, genders, sexualities, ethnicity, and classes as "other." As migrants in the United States, our native lands, our *costumbres* (customs), native *lengua* (language), and familias are devalued and seen as morally bankrupt. Navigating new spaces and experiencing ourselves within multiple and new identities has shaped who we are and who we want to be in this new land.

Natalia is a political refugee from Colombia who came to the United States escaping multiple violences—drug wars, civil war, gendered violence, and displacement. Mónica grew up in the northern part of Spain, Galicia: a land of immigrants. Mónica left Spain under a very different sociopolitical reality than her family members before her. Those sociopolitical transformations allowed Mónica to access higher education and leave her country with a university degree. She immigrated to the Netherlands, where she lived for several years, working at different blue-collar jobs until she mastered the language, after which she ended up working as a counselor. She left the Netherlands and moved to the United States, following her partner's career. It was a journey of *sacrificios* (sacrifices) for the sake of the familia. It was a journey of learned experiences and multiple lessons on what it means to be an immigrant: the separations; the encounters with the unfamiliar; the state of being an outsider, of living in between two worlds and developing a new sense of identity and trying to find a place where to belong.

We both attended graduate school in the United States, in sociology and psychology, respectively. Entering the United States through the doors of graduate school gave us access to a better understanding of what education means in this country and introduced us to a venue to start action in different spaces. Natalia experienced the circumstances of being the only Latinx woman in her graduate program and having a constant reminder of who she was. Mónica attended graduate school in the field of psychology, working as a clinician, and learned the reality of an educational system made for the privileged ones, institutions that oppress and impose on individuals without considering the devastating impact this has on their well-being.

We were both penalized for being outspoken, for being political, for being different, for being "too passionate," "too enthusiastic," and "too direct"; there was something about us that made some people uncomfortable, but others trusted and confided in us. These encounters and experiences exhausted and frustrated us, but at other times they were opportunities for us to clarify what we wanted to do with our knowledge, with our "beings." We realized the importance in this society of identifying and positioning yourself, as well as marking and treating others differently depending on their accent and their phenotypic characteristics, especially their skin color.

Chicana/o Department "Comunidad" at UC Davis

Most of the students in the Department of Chicana/o Studies identify as female (82%) and 100% are between the ages of eighteen and twenty-seven years old. The great majority are first-generation (96%) and have been at the university for more than one year (94%) (West 2017, 42). Many of the students depend on financial assistance to persist in higher education. Of the fifty students who responded, 96% indicated that they currently relied on grants, while 60% of the students relied upon loans to help finance their education (44). In addition, the majority (78%) are employed and work ten to thirty hours per week (44–45). In "Exploration of the Prevalence and Experiences of Low-Income Latinx Undergraduate Students Navigating Food and Housing Insecurity at a Four-Year Research University," Alyssa West (2017) concluded that for those UC Davis Chicana/o Studies students who had completed the survey, food insecurity (11%), housing instability (17%), and homelessness (6%) were issues impacting success and well-being. Institutional barriers, along with the lack of resources or awareness of resources (both on and off campus), likely contribute to poorer academic and health outcomes (West, 46–53).

In our interactions with students, we acknowledge the psychological implications of the daily challenges that they face and the importance of caring for them. We see the benefit of a classroom environment where they are validated, they feel they belong, and they are safe.

We have a holistic understanding of our students' needs, and in our roles, we treat them each as a whole person; we encourage them to be who they are. We invite them to express their multiple identities without feeling shame. Our work is in collaboration with them because we learn from them; they inspire us; they give meaning to what we do; they consider us their mentors, advocates, allies, and *tías* (aunts). The students see us crying when we witness injustices and the pain is too intense, but they also see us laughing and celebrating life. Our students share their experiences; they come to our offices to ask for help and for guidance. We hear stories of pain, trauma, persecution, sexual assaults, and losses. The students recognize us when helping them and their peers to find resources, staff, faculty, or offices. Students see us as part of *la comunidad* of the Department of Chicana/o Studies, a welcoming and safe environment within UC Davis. We have developed a network of people on campus who we know are there to help and support; we connect students with them, and we can say that *cada día son más* (every day there are more), thanks to the work of previous generations of professors, staff members who *sembraron* (sowed) the ground for changes. We want students to experience a learning environment where they feel they belong, to let them know that they matter and that they have the right to express and be. We want students to bring their knowledge, their families, their narratives, their thinking; we want them to go into their communities or other communities and use their knowledge to change realities; we want them to move from passive receivers into active participants. We want all students to be part of a common learning experience based on solidarity, understanding, *respecto* (respect), and care for others as well. We want to give what is not given as an act of care and social justice within academia and the larger society. We hear all the hardships they encounter; we are aware that supporting them goes beyond individual efforts and that we need the community. We know that many students will give up their academic journey if we, as community, are not there for them. Also, it is too much pain, sorrow, and *angustia* (concern) to bear alone.

Unfortunately, our offices must always have available tissue boxes, both for students and for us. As Latina faculty we share with them how we navigate our own academic institutions so that students can draw on cultural knowledge and skills to foster academic and social counterspaces in which to build culturally supportive communities. As Latina faculty we battle to balance demands of research, teaching, mentorship, and service work (Joseph and Hirshfield

2011). As Latina faculty we receive a disproportionate number of requests to mentor and to do service. As faculty we are tapped to serve on numerous committees for our "unique perspective." The individual attention that, as Latina faculty, we are willing to provide is an unrecognized cornerstone in efforts to create a sense of belonging and to retain our students at UC Davis. Our invisible labor has been described as cultural taxation (Padilla 1994): the pressure Latina faculty feel to serve as role models, mentors, and proxy parents to Latinx and Chicanx students, and to meet all institutional needs. As Latina faculty we mentor and advise current and former Latinx and Chicanx undergraduate students in our major and in other majors. Most of them are first-generation students who need extra support to navigate college life. We also advise and mentor Latinx and Chicanx graduate students who need support in applying to and navigating graduate school. As Latina faculty we intercede on behalf of students and try to educate colleagues on the nuances of gender-based, race-based, class-based, and nationality-based issues that impact the lives of our students (Hirshfield and Joseph 2012). We advise and help not only Latinx students but all students who take our classes and need support.

Our students honor us by sharing how they ended up under academic probation or being subject to dismissal. Listening to their experiences and how easily they got into these situations forces us to actively advocate for, mentor, support, and guide them. We are involved in providing this advocacy, support, and guidance as an act of resistance to an institution that seems to be operating to make Chicanx and Latinx students fail. As faculty, we openly question the administration: How does UC Davis, which makes great efforts to recruit Latinx and Chicanx students, end up having such dismal push-out rates? We openly express our concerns at the lack of Chicanx and Latinx faculty and staff who represent the Latinx and Chicanx students. We are aware of the difficulties that students face, and we hear their experiences of being rejected, silenced, misadvised, misguided, and denigrated by racist and discriminatory comments in interactions with different members of the UC Davis community. As faculty we discuss and plan how to implement in our courses practices that promote a sense of belonging and develop strategies that embrace an inclusive model within academia where we all "belong." Our classes promote critical thinking, encourage social action, and stimulate activism by teaching students the power young people, mothers, and other common folk have always had to build solidarity and promote collective action and social justice movements for equity. We act as caring agents for them by promoting alliances, connecting them with resources, and inspiring them to use their resilience, knowledge, and cultural and family heritage to overcome the difficulties and resist.

We, as Chicana feminists, reclaim care as an act of social justice, particularly in the work we do in the context of academia. We experience the explicit patriarchal violent environment where care is delegated to ethnic studies departments and their faculty or staff who are often women of color. The result of this alienation of caregivers serves a function to the others who do not carry the burden. As Professor Chabram mentioned in a conversation, "Others can exist thanks to the feminization of caregivers in the context of Chican/o/x studies." We end by calling for a feminist university, a university that acknowledges our labor and our efforts toward the creation of belonging and of safe spaces on campus in spite of the racist and antiracist discourse and systemic policies that are in place and affect our students. We call for a feminist university that recognizes that it takes all our energy, *ganas* (desire), and *coraje* (courage) for our classes to be safe spaces that humanize the learning experience, create solidarity with students, and model what we would like to see become the norm: acceptance, respect, and tolerance.

References

Cervantes-Soon, Claudia, and Juan Carrillo. 2016. "Toward a Pedagogy of Border Thinking: Building on Latin@ Students' Subaltern Knowledge." *High School Journal* 99 (4): 282–301.

Davis, Angela Y. 2012. "Social Justice in the Public University of California: Reflections and Strategies." Speech given during a teach-in at the University of California, Davis, February 23, 2012.

Delgado Bernal, Dolores. 2001. "Learning and Living Pedagogies of the Home: The Mestiza Consciousness of Chicana Students." *International Journal of Qualitative Studies in Education* 14 (5): 623–39.

Dyrness, Andrea. 2011. *Mothers United: An Immigrant Struggle for Socially Just Education.* Minneapolis: University of Minnesota Press.

Flores, Yvette. 2015. *Psychology Perspectives for the Chicano and Latino Family.* San Diego: Cognella, Academic Publishing, 2015.

Freire, Paulo. 1970. *Pedagogy of the Oppressed.* Translated by Myra Bergman Ramos. New York: Continuum.

Hirshfield, Laura E., and Tiffany D. Joseph. 2012. "'We Need a Woman, We Need a Black Woman': Gender, Race, and Identity Taxation in the Academy." *Gender and Education* 24, no. 2: 213–27.

Joseph, Tiffany D., and Laura E. Hirshfield. 2011. "'Why Don't You Get Somebody New to Do It?' Race and Cultural Taxation in the Academy." *Ethnic and Racial Studies* 34 (1): 121–41.

Lara, Irene. 2013. "Healing Sueños for Academia." In *This Bridge We Call Home: Radical Visions for Transformation*, edited by Gloria Anzaldúa and AnaLouise Keating, 447–52. New York: Routledge.

Lee, John. 2013. "What Do Butterflies Have to Do with Open Borders? Migration Is Beautiful." Open Borders (blog). May 27, 2013. https://openborders.info/blog/what-do-butterflies-have-to-do-with-open-borders-migration-is-beautiful/.

Oliveira, Gabriella. 2018. *Motherhood Across Borders: Immigrants and their Children in Mexico and New York*. New York: New York University Press.

Padilla, Amado M. 1994. "Ethnic Minority Scholars, Research, and Mentoring: Current and Future Issues." *Educational Researcher* 23(4): 24–27.

West, Alyssa. 2017. "The Struggle Is Real: Exploration of the Prevalence and Experiences of Low-Income Latinx Undergraduate Students Navigating Food and Housing Insecurity at a Four-Year Research University." Unpublished master's thesis, CSU Sacramento. https://csu-csus.esploro.exlibrisgroup.com/esploro/outputs/graduate/The-struggle-is-real--an/99257830875301671.

CHAPTER 11

Radical Self-Care

MARIA R. PALACIOS

Maria R. Palacios's contribution provides a much-needed retort to notions of self-care that permeate health media. These media often fault patients for their own burnout and promote individualistic solutions. In contrast, Palacios calls for a relational community engagement. Her contribution talks back to generalized universal renditions of self-care through a poetic means that grounds this practice in the experiences and insights of the chronicle of a disabled Latina. Palacios advocates for herself and for others and suggests that self-care involves responding forcefully to widely held social generalizations about the disabled. Key to her vision is the idea that self-care is akin to education and community literacy. Finally, she supports a testimonial vision of self-care, as this education cannot exist if disabled people don't bear witness to their afflictions, victories, and experiences with the medical establishment as well as to their multiple connections to society.

To the disabled, self-care means
surviving
surviving poverty,
surviving ignorance,

Excerpt. The whole piece appears on Maria R. Palacio's blog and was recently published on OPEN DOORS (https://www.opendoorsnyc.org/freestyle-friday/guest-speaker-art) with minor edits.

surviving segregation,
surviving
the invisibility forced upon our lives.

To the disabled, self-care means making sure
we don't die
of hunger,
we don't die of sadness,
we don't die alone, abandoned, and forgotten
in some shithole nursing home
that paints a peaceful transition to heaven
but is a living hell behind closed doors.

Self-care means we force open the doors
that were made to imprison us.
It means breaking the oppressing chains
that hold disabled people down
and acknowledging that none of us can move up
when others are still down.

We must keep each other alive while the nondisabled world
wants us to die, disappear, become extinct,
a thing of the past, at last, eliminating
the infirm, the broken,
the undesirable.

Self-care means unlearning the bullshit we've been told
about our disabled bodies, the lies we've been forced to wear
in nondisabled costume,
like Blackface, forcing us to try to fake
able-bodiedness we do not have,
finding humor in our struggles
while feeling ashamed of our differences.

Self-care means we learn to love our differences
and recognize

that we have our personal greatness as a gift.
It means we know how others lift
our bodies like heavy crosses they must bear
while we endure the pain of their ableist fears.

For the disabled, self-care means we undress our own fears
knowing that doing so will hurt.
It means letting others know the hurt
caused by their actions,
caused by ableist words casually thrown
to describe our bodies.

Self-care means we forgive our bodies
for not walking, not talking, not seeing,
not hearing, not thinking, not acting,
not feeling, not being
like the boring *normals* who think they're better.

Self-care means a better understanding
of our right to exist,
our right to resist, our right
to love ourselves without guilt.
Self-care means
we forgive those who trespass
against our rights
but do so by making sure it doesn't happen again.

Self-care means knowing
it will happen again, and again
and again,
and knowing we will again
and again go back
to the battlefield
to slay the dragons of ableist crap
that trap
disabled people

into believing that the normies know,
more than we do,
about our bodies and our needs.

Self-care means *we* get to explain our needs
to the doctors, to the attendants,
to the social workers, to the concerned relatives,
to the "professionals" who think they're experts at living our lives.

Self-care means remembering all that
when the only thing we can remember
is the past-due bill on the table
and the fear of not being able to make ends meet
this month, or the next, or the next.
Self-care means telling ourselves that next time
will be different,
although we're not sure how.

Self-care means we know how
to survive because it's something
we've simply learned to do.
Self-care means asking for help knowing it's OK to ask.
It means asking for help
and asking exactly for what we need
and without feeling guilty for it.

Self-care means remembering
that we don't have to apologize for our needs.
Self-care, to us, means allowing our wounds
to heal out in the open.
It means knowing we don't have to cover up our pain,
nor do we have to disclose it
in order to validate our truths.

Self-care means our relationship with pain,
like our relationship with God, is personal.

Self-care, when we're disabled, means
learning to self-regulate positivity because
the nondisabled world only sees negativity and pity
instead of strength and love.

Self-care means we are aware of our personal strengths
but also know we don't always have to be strong.
Self-care means letting the tears flow in order to heal the soul.
Self-care means we know it is the soul
through which we exist in our bodies.
It means we love our bodies
but are fully aware of how fragile they can be . . .

Self-care means . . .
we own our bodies even
when the medical model's broken definition of who we are
may say otherwise, because when we're disabled,
owning our bodies is the most radical form of self-care and self-love
we will ever practice and exercise,
and it will be the most criticized and
revolutionary action of our lives, and the nondisabled
will continue to fight for the right to live for us
while we exist in our nonnormative bodies
and our nonconforming minds.
Society whines at the outcry of our rebellious advocacy,
but rebellious advocacy is
how we practice self-care.

We practice self-care
by constantly performing CPR on our broken dreams,
by remembering that others will forget us
because they always forget about us
although they pretended to remember us
during the evacuation drill
where fake disabled people played our part
and real disabled people were left behind because . . . well . . .

we must never forget
that others will not remember
but they will always remember to tell us what to do
and how to live.

When we're disabled,
self-care also involves telling nondisabled people to back off
and fuck off, if we must go to that extreme.
Self-care, when we're disabled, sometimes requires extreme
measures
like acknowledging the pleasures often denied to us
in the name of normality.

Self-care involves the beautiful abnormality
of crip-sexy
and the way we define sexy
and claim the power of our bodies
as the wholeness that makes us complete.

Self-care means
we don't have to compete to be less disabled
in order to prove our worth.
Self-care means we know we are worth the chance . . .
the chance to love,
the chance to share,
the chance to be part of the world that fears us . . .

Self-care means having to remind ourselves
that disability never equals
the devaluing of our lives and our right to exist
and to make community within a community of our choice.

Self-care means we know we have a choice
and a right to choose
and nobody has the right to use
our differences as an excuse for the denial
of our human rights.

When we're disabled, self-care means
constantly educating others
about our basic rights,
always repeating ourselves
and our realities out of mere necessity
because if we don't,
the nondisabled world will pretend we don't exist.
Self-care means we resist.
We say yes.
We say no.
We own every aspect of our lives even
when every aspect of our lives may depend
on nondisabled assistance.
It means we project our power from within,
letting the normies know
they don't have the right to decide for us
unless we give them permission to do so . . .

It means we say "enough" when it's been too much,
and we do it without hesitation
because we know we have the right to say *enough.*
Enough ableist lies.
Enough ignorant remarks.
Enough pity-loaded amens.
Enough expectations of inspiration.
We do not owe you space
in our personal space
simply because we may not fit
your boring definition of normalcy . . .

Self-care means we sustain and support one another.
We lift each other up,
knowing
that unless we do,
we *will* be forgotten.
We repeat this in our heads
over and over because otherwise, we, too, can forget.

Ableism is always lurking,
looking for a way in,
knocking on the door of our crip identity,
trying to make us forget
that we have the right to be ourselves
in our personal liberation, in our definition of self
and whatever liberation means to us
as disabled people
with our own extensions
of, often, half-narrated sections
of truths we are still learning about ourselves
because being disabled is just one aspect of who we are . . .

Self-care means we retell our stories
until they get it right,
until our voices are heard,
and until the various parts of who we are
become evident to ourselves
and to those who negate our positive crip identity.

Self-care means being proud of our differences,
embracing our uniqueness,
celebrating our power,
knowing that while some are fighting
for the right to bear arms,
disabled people are still fighting
for the right to bear life,
for the right to exist and the right to see ourselves
in future generations . . .

Self-care means
trying to find the time to rest
while the world thinks that
being disabled means that rest
is all we get all the time because we are broken
and can't work

or contribute or find success as is it measured
by capitalism.

Self-care means learning to survive capitalism
through solidarity and the sustainability of hope
because it is only when we are there for one another
that somebody will be there for us
when the time comes for us to survive . . .

Those of us who have been there already know that.
We stand by the entrance of the temple
calling others to the table,
teaching the new ones
that that they're able to move on, to reach out,
to realize that the light is not out
although darkness is real.

Self-care is about survival.
When we're disabled,
self-care is, always, about survival.
It's about economic justice,
food justice,
sex justice,
social justice,
and making sure the movement
and the march don't move on without us
because unless we are there to remind them, they will
move on
without us.

Self-care, when we're disabled,
is a nonstop advocacy ride,
and until we are no longer oppressed by ableism,
self-care will continue to be just another definition
of privilege.

CHAPTER 12

"Dis-ease" in Academia Is Not a Secret

A Meditation on Caregiving

INÉS HERNÁNDEZ-ÁVILA

In this essay Inés Hernández-Ávila vividly describes how devastating academia can be for a woman professor of color in academia, by analyzing her experiences as a successful Native woman senior scholar in Native American studies who is on the verge of retiring. Her career has spanned Native American and Indigenous studies as well as Chicanx studies and has been filled with achievement and accomplishment, but also with grief, anxiety, and torment, which have often caused illness. She writes with both a sense of outrage and a sense of urgency and hope, sharing strategies to activate support and communities in academia.

I.

Soy una mujer de palabra
Mis padres me enseñaron
lo que vale mi voz.
Mi palabra surge
desde el centro
de mi ser
mi corazón
mi luzespíritu
siempre.

I write as a woman professor of color in academia. I am a Nimiipuu/Tejana feminist senior scholar, poet, and visual artist in Native American studies, on the verge of retiring. In a way, it is a kind of exit reflection that I am compelled to write, about how devastatingly unhealthy academia can be for faculty from underrepresented communities, with a focus on Native American / Indigenous and Chicana/o/e faculty because these are the communities I know best.

I offer this meditation to bring to the foreground the sometimes blatant, sometimes subtle ways the academic-industrial complex infringes on our humanity, our dignity, and our worth and seeks to sustain its racialized, gendered, white supremacist, heteropatriarchal hierarchy. I write as a response to the question, How do we heal from the assaults of academia on our beings? First, we help each other to diagnose the dis-ease, the wounds, the harm, the slights, the batterings, and we name them. In the naming, we release the intrusions into our spaces and begin to heal. We reclaim our breath, our health, our voice, and our presence. In doing so, we return to our powers, including the power to self-heal and to heal others. In this sense, this meditation is a call to care work, or gift giving to self and to others.

I am inclined to think there are many stories that need to be told, heard, and acknowledged—and yet, often, we self-silence for a complex number of reasons. As my colleague Angie Chabram has said, "We are ailing and if the dis-ease is not addressed, if the stories are not spoken, they will fester."[1] We must tell the stories, and as the late poet Karenne Wood says in her poem "The Poet I Wish I Was," "We can't change the beginning or the middle—we can only try to rewrite the end" (2018, 237). Or, as Gloria Anzaldúa has written, "To change or reinvent reality, you engage the facultad of your imagination . . . Imagination opens the road to both personal and societal change—transformation of self, consciousness, community, society" (2015, 44). I firmly believe that in the ethnic studies programs, this is the work being done.

My career has spanned Native American and Indigenous studies and Chicanx studies. It has been a life challenge to be in the academy. I have been successful (I am one of a small number of Native women who are full professors in the country), and I'm happy with my achievements, the positive

1. Email communication to me from Prof. Angie Chabram, November 1, 2022.

experiences I've lived as a faculty member, and the good colleagues on my campus whom I have met and befriended over the years. At the same time, my path has been filled with grief, anxiety, and torment, which have caused illness in my being. My lens is quite personal, and my story arises from both a sense of outrage and a sense of urgency and hope. I write about what I have lived through, what I have witnessed, what individuals have shared with me, and what strategies have come to me to activate protection, support, and healing, for myself and other underrepresented individuals and communities in academia. My primary attention here is principally on faculty in the ethnic studies programs. A focus on students (undergraduate and graduate) would be another story, although these stories are intertwined and must be told also.

I have witnessed much in Western institutions of higher learning, in particular as they impact the communities I consider to be mine; in other words, the communities to which I belong. I have a keen eye and a sound memory. My institutional memory spans more than three decades. This bearing of witness is, in some ways, a breaking of silence. What I have to say might be applicable to other communities of color and all those who are underserved by the academy in this society. I also know there are others whose voices have been heard on this subject. I join my voices to theirs.

II.

A matter of life and death: *On February 10, 2022, I almost died. I literally looked death in the face and almost left this earth. I think of Audre Lorde's "The Transformation of Silence into Language and Action," remembering how she begins that essay writing that she faced a scare with cancer, and how this turn of events gave her pause (2007, 40). I am currently in a pause mode, reflecting on my life, allowing myself to feel and be illuminated by what I have lived.*

I am humbled that I have been allowed a reprieve. It is not yet my time. Was this a wake-up call? Yes. Yes. In this pause mode (which is a slowing down), I am (finally) contemplating, deeply, the way I have dedicated my life to academia, to building Native American studies, and before this, in Texas, Mexican American studies. I have said often that I have given blood to the Native American Studies program at UC Davis, where I have been for more than thirty years. With what Lorde called "harsh and urgent clarity" (2007, 40), I know that my own health issues mostly have to do with life in academia. In my personal spaces I am content and fulfilled.

In the midst of my life crisis, a dear friend succumbed to cancer, a warrior woman and ardent feminist who is beloved by so many of us throughout the country and beyond: Beatriz Pesquera. I first met her in the 1980s, when I arrived at UC Davis as a lecturer. She was already on tenure track in Chicana/o Studies, and she was a builder of the program. We became close friends, confidantes, accomplices—we both loved, loved, loved to dance, to laugh, to *comadrear*, to discuss ideas. I love(d) her so much, as did my mom, my sons, and my husband. She was/is family. She used to say we needed to create T-shirts for those of us who were/are daring, rebellious women, T-shirts with "*Brujas de Aztlán*" blazoned on the front. She was one of the leading activists of the Third World liberation movement in the Bay Area. She went on one of the earliest Venceremos Brigade trips to Cuba, and she continued her support of Cuba throughout her life. She was both a sought-after professor and an extremely capable administrator.

"Sufro la imensa pena de tu extravío / Siento el dolor profundo de tu partida."[2] Beatriz, like many of our generation, came to academia as an activist. We were passionately engaged in social struggle on many fronts, and academia quickly became another front, perhaps the most crucial of them all, because in academia we were/are engaging in the dismantling of those systemic and disciplinary frameworks that for so long perpetuated assessments of our communities that were hostile, belittling, and outright racist. In our programs, we are constantly breaking the silences and articulating for ourselves our assessments of the issues pertaining to our communities. Indeed, these programs came about because of a collective *"Ya basta!"* to academia for presuming to dissect us, pathologize us, criminalize us, explain away our "inability" to progress, and render us less than human. In Native American studies, Chicana/o studies, Asian American studies, and African and African American studies, our courses provide a way for our peoples to be seen for their strengths, their creativity, their envisioning, their agency/protagonism—and this dynamic and these teachings are healing for all of us, on the campus and beyond. It is painful to the core, then, when dissension emerges from these very programs.

2. As sung by Bebo Valdés and Diego el Cigala in "Lágrimas Negras."

Beatriz faced some painfully disheartening slights from one of her own colleagues right before she decided to retire early. Seeing how she was treated was devastating and almost unreal. It was sickening. And yet she bravely pushed forward—she had an incredibly high *aguante,* as we would say in Spanish. Many of us know what this means—to be able to withstand whatever is tossed at you, to know how to deflect, to know how to keep standing strong, *no matter what.*

As I rest from almost dying, I keep entering into reveries
where memories (re)present themselves to me
flowing through me in spontaneously coherent clusters
apparently disparate moments suddenly pass
before my eyes and I understand

III.

En algo nos parecemos, luna de mi soledad.
Yo voy cantando y penando
Es mi modo de alumbrar.
Atahualpa Yupanqui

From the beginning: When I did my job talk at UC Davis, I also had to meet with each member of the search committee one on one. When I met with the external (white) member of the committee, he told me, point blank, "The strongest thing you have going for you is that you know who you are. The institution will do everything in its power to take that away from you. Don't let it." He was right. The unspoken but palpably felt message from academia is to blend in, to be like everyone else, to think, dress, speak like everyone else, which means privileging the West, always, especially the criteria by which a person and her/his/their work are interpreted and evaluated.

When I went up for full professor, I was at first turned down. The message I received, along with the split vote, said, literally, that my "moral and cultural commitment [was] a hindrance to [my] career." I couldn't believe my eyes when I read that statement. The message rose up from the page to engrave itself on my forehead. Fortunately, my department responded quickly, as did I, and the decision was reversed. But that statement has stayed with me because it reveals to me that the reviewing committee *saw* this commitment, even though they disparaged it. I am actually quite proud that they *got me.* Some of them might not have approved of me or my work, but they got me enough to see my *compromiso* and to let me know that, from their perspective, this compromiso would not serve me well in academia. How dare they?

I am currently one of four Native American faculty on the Davis campus, and we are all in Native American Studies. When I retire, there will be three. This makes us almost invisible, since the university is so obsessed with numbers. Numbers are what count in a corporatized university.

IV.

Microaggressions—vignettes: I have been the target of bullying, and I have witnessed bullying in academia—a bullying that often gets rewarded rather than punished or even reprimanded. Once, in conversation with a dean about a troublesome colleague, the dean responded, "Oh, but [this person] does so well with the donors!" And that ended that. Numbers again. This time in dollars.

I have witnessed colleagues getting pushed out of mainstream departments only to find a home in an ethnic studies department, where, by the way, these individuals have flourished. The mainstream departments evidently have preordained criteria for who passes muster, and people of color rarely are seen to meet those criteria.

I have witnessed an incredibly gifted senior scholar (at another University of California campus) be held back from becoming full professor by her mainstream department even though she created a specialty area pertaining to Native American studies in her program and mentored and hooded a majority of the scholars now working in this particular subfield of Native American and Indigenous studies. What is heartbreaking is that her department finally promoted her to full professor, but they waited so long to do so that she passed away soon after. The story of how this scholar was not valued by her program, even though the scholar's reputation is international, is a chilling one that caused deep pain and outrage to those colleagues who know what an amazing leader she was in her field and how her contributions live on in all those she mentored.

I have witnessed younger colleagues pretend that they do not need their senior faculty. In fact, they engage in name-calling and behave as if the work of the senior faculty is irrelevant, that they are the ones "in the know," that their perspectives are what matter most. It is almost amusing, but not—the senior faculty are the ones who hired the younger colleagues—which means the senior faculty valued their work and had great hopes for them as colleagues. I have also witnessed senior faculty who are dismayed and disheartened by this turn of events.[3] For those of us in ethnic studies programs, this was never what we imagined. Our programs were created from the ground up, from protests, from demands to institutions of higher learning that spaces be opened for us to create disciplinary fields of study pertaining to our communities, *in our own ways and on our own terms.* The building of an academic program, from this perspective, is also intimately related to community building for our respective peoples. When envisioning our fields, we engage(d) in inter-, multi-, and transdisciplinary theorizing, decolonizing methodologies, and radical pedagogies, for the benefit of our students and our communities and to rewrite and re-right the scholarly record of what counts as authoritative expertise regarding our communities.

It seemed a given that we would do our best to engage with each other as autonomous individuals working toward collective autonomies for the distinct communities that we serve. In other words, it has always behooved us to act in principled ways with each other because the stakes are so high—the faculty in our programs are serving as thought leaders to create social transformation and social justice in this society—our programs must be protected. From cultural perspectives, presumably we know how important it is to be *buena gente*, to show respect. This ideal often seems long gone these days. It is difficult to sustain the mantra of community, when in our daily work lives, "community" seems more of a fanciful fiction, or worse, an empty notion. The disjuncture between what has become codified as sacred in our programs—the idea of community, and community building—and how this principle is expressed and practiced can become jarring and contribute to personal and collective dis-ease.

I remember one time, a long while ago, after a particularly heated departmental discussion about some topic or the other, one of my colleagues blurted out "But we're all family!" which was said to beseech us to not argue. My response at the time? "We are not a family. I have a family; I've experi-

3. Unfortunately, I have also heard of senior faculty who evidently see themselves as gatekeepers and hold up the promotion process for faculty junior to them in ethnic studies programs.

enced family dysfunction—I don't want any more in any other kind of family. To me, what we are is a community—of scholars, students, staff—and as a community we should always remember to show each other respect." In the private space of a family, sometimes dysfunction is simply ignored or tolerated. In a community, a collective awareness is a must and has the potential of nurturing relationships and the promise of incredible futurities among us. The idea of thinking of ourselves as a community is the recognition of each other's autonomy and that we don't all have to be each other's best friends. As individuals, we have our circles of communities that are dear to us—we need to respect the fact that each of us has a life beyond academia, and many of those aspects are private, intimate. This, however, does not preclude us forming friendships and collegial relationships with each other at work, as members of the community in the programs to which we belong, and it may be that those friendships become long lasting outside of academia. For me, the idea of family seems to create a set of expectations to which we may or may not agree, but the idea of community serves as an invitation of belonging in a professional space.

The spaces of encounter: One arena of struggle is within our departments. Another, our relationships with other departments and the campus as a whole. Another, our relationships with our students. Another, our collaborative relationships with other colleagues. Another, the entire area of service (departmental, campus, system—in the case of the University of California campuses—professional, public/community). We are constantly negotiating, navigating our way through academia. It behooves us to pay attention, to notice everything, *for our own well-being.* In each of these spaces, our voices are resounding in their silent reverberations that seep through into our daily lived spaces—enough so that we (our bodies, our hearts, our spirits, our minds) feel something is wrong, but we don't always know how to name what we're feeling, since the details, the stories, are hidden in secrecy. These are the stories we must hear to be able to help ourselves release them.

V.

The university's duplicity: Ironically, our university has a Principles of Community statement, but in many cases, I have seen flagrant violations of these principles by some faculty, through outright bullying (yelling, name-calling, physical intimidation, verbal abuse, disrespect, invasion of a person's space by the abuser's coming too close in a threatening manner), or through seemingly more subtle forms of bullying—what in Spanish we would call *indirectas*, insinuating comments or actions that are not quite addressed explicitly to anyone, and yet the person on the receiving end of an *indirecta* often knows the comment or action was directed at them.

Bullying is one of the major causes for dis-ease in academia. And bullies, when they are called on their behavior, often turn around and lie by accusing the one bullied of being the aggressor. They love to play the victim when it suits them. If there are bullies in a small program (such as the ethnic studies programs), the resultant tension and overflow of toxicity can irrevocably damage the ambience of the entire department, creating obstacles to the free engagement of ideas, the respectful sharing of our work, and the possibility of joy in each other's accomplishments.

The consequence of such a situation is an unhealthy work environment, in which individuals dread going to meetings and avoid speaking up for fear of being ridiculed or insulted. Or, just as bad, departmental meetings glaze over the toxicity, and colleagues participate with an odd form of civility that occludes any sign or vestige of toxicity by simply moving on without comment. The emotional/psychological damage may not appear to affect everyone, but as with all forms of violation, those who see, hear, or know of aggressive behavior are left with the feelings that the violence caused to the whole. In such situations, any collective action toward enhancing these programs becomes almost impossible to achieve.

Toxicity in academia has not gone unnoticed. In the *Times Higher Education* issue of November 2019, in an article titled "Ten Rules for Succeeding in Academia Through Upward Toxicity," the author, Irina Dumitrescu, notes the following:

> Universities sing the song of meritocracy but dance to a different tune. In reality, they will do everything to reward and protect their most destructive, abusive and uncooperative faculty. The more thoroughly such scholars poison departments, programmes and individual lives, the more universities double down to please them.

In many instances it seems that when a faculty member's accomplishments bring prestige or money to the university, everything else is conveniently unnoticed. The university basically says yes to money and prestige, *at whatever cost*, so in effect, bullies are protected, though they are the cause of so much damage and heartache.

VI.

Yo no le canto a la luna
porque alumbra y nada más
Le canto porque ella sabe de mi largo caminar
le canto porque ella sabe
de mi largo caminar.
—Atahualpa Yupanqui

The disregard of our work by academia: I have perceived how the institution views fields such as ethnic studies, Chicanx studies, Native American and Indigenous studies, Asian American studies, and African and African American studies. To me, the more recently instituted offices of diversity, equity, and inclusion (DEI) are meant to contain and control any issues having to do with people of color. These offices of diversity, equity, and inclusion never deign to consult with the specialists who work in the above fields. The institution of DEI offices is another way that we are marginalized, if not erased, on our campuses. The irony is that we are not blind or unaware; on the contrary, we observe closely this ignoring of our fields. In contrast, I remember how, years ago, I read the UCSC equivalent of the UC Davis magazine. The UCSC cover story was about the Latin American and Latino Studies program and how the faculty in this program are "thought leaders." I immediately sent this story to our administration, noting that it would be a grand day if Davis ever did anything similar.

Beyond Davis, I have been a mentor to many scholars who stay in touch with me. I have heard horror stories about the overwhelming pressures of life in academia. It doesn't stop even after an individual has become a tenured faculty member. I recently saw a younger tenured colleague at a conference in Texas; she mentioned to me that she had to leave one position to take another because of extreme stress-related issues on her former campus that resulted in a grievous health crisis for her. In April 2022 I received an email message from a dear colleague, Margo Tamez, Lipan Apache, gifted poet and associate professor of Indigenous Studies at the University of British Columbia. She wrote to share the report of the University of British Columbia president's Anti-Racism and Inclusive Excellence Task Force, 2021–22, and to let me know that she had participated as a task force member, providing her lived and felt experiences to the report. She states in her email that she reached out to me because I have consistently supported her, saying,

> You have helped me to process the numerous difficult and often dangerous acts of anti-Indigenous racism, misogyny, homophobia, sexism, ableism, and anti-Indigenous Americas sentiment in my academic journey. You have helped me process and comprehend the systemic and structural factors which have inhibited, contained, walled, diminished and trivialized my numerous complaints against academic oppressors.[4]

Professor Tamez is not one to mince words, in her scholarship or in her poetry. Hers is a fierce courage, and she will not be silenced. What is her saving grace? That she can reach out to those of us who support her to remind herself that she is not alone. She has a network that is international in scope. Sadly, though, that doesn't mean that she can rely on this distant support, when on the ground, in her daily work, as a scholar, professor/poet, activist, and visionary, she still must deal with the systemic and structural factors she referenced. The same is true for any of us in similar situations. And yes, we need to stand with each other, even across long distances, because it is the way we hold each other up. It is the way we heal each other.

When an individual is in a mainstream department/program, there is not so much program building, since mainstream fields have been in place for centuries. In the newer area-studies programs, which include the ethnic studies programs; American studies; women, gender, and sexuality studies; queer studies; and disability studies, the faculty have the task of program building (and therefore visioning), the task of ensuring the prestige and status of these fields, and the task of making said prestige and status markedly visible in academia, especially on one's own campus. The building of prestige of a program ensures the prestige accorded to the faculty. Everything comes full circle. Here is where faculty, in thinking of themselves as a community—as an activist community in struggle to create transformation—will, or can, hopefully, see the need for collective action, for consensus (which is next

4. Margo Tamez, email communication to me, April 22, 2022.

to impossible when faculty disregard or ignore each other and prefer to act as individuals with no obligation to the program that hired them).

VII.

Useful strategies to thwart the academy's attempts on our well-being: In Native American studies, I had exceptional mentors, namely David Risling Jr., Sarah Hutchison, George Longfish, and, at times, Jack Forbes. They were my elders, and I am forever appreciative of their guidance, their protection, their humor, and their love. I have other wonderful colleagues as well, some now retired, who are/were my trusted confidants. These colleagues are spread across the country, the hemisphere, and the globe.

To heal we have to first see and feel the problems, contemplate them, and decide, by whatever means, how to address them. One teaching I received from George Longfish, Seneca/Tuscarora artist, emeritus professor of Native American Studies, and healer: "When a combustible issue comes up in a faculty meeting, or in any other space, pull your energy completely out of everything, and just observe. You don't have to do a thing. Just watch." This is incredibly useful advice; often, for faculty of color, we might feel that we must respond immediately in particular situations or settings. This disengagement allows a space to breathe, to consider what is being said or done, to observe the complexities of a given problem, to not give in to reacting quickly.

Another major teaching I received from David Risling Jr. (Hupa, Yurok, Karok), one of the founders of Native American Studies at Davis, is this: "Pick your battles. And once you pick them, prepare for them. Go into battle knowing that you're going to win." Easily enough said, and wise, but sometimes tricky to accomplish. For those of us who come from underserved communities, communities that are called "marginalized," when we enter academia, we often don't trust the institution. It is an unfamiliar space, especially if we are first generation. In such a space of unknowingness, we have to learn how the system works, and we "suspicion" a lot (to use Craig Womack's [2010] transformation of the term from a noun to a verb). In our suspicionings, we can tend to see patterns of inequality and outright discrimination fairly easily. But as many of us have learned, we do have to choose when and how to respond, as David Risling Jr. indicated. This does take a toll on us, however, because when we pick one battle over another, we have to live with what we chose to endure without response. These instances when we (have to) choose *not to respond* leave an energy that creates a lingering illness, an un-ease we carry with us. We have to learn how to release, release, release any energy that causes distress and dis-ease.

I remember being subjected to the whims of some faculty during my time here at Davis, not so much recently, but when I was a fresh full professor and began to sit on major Academic Senate committees. One individual (a fellow committee member) accosted me rudely at a formal dinner to celebrate a colleague's retirement. His intention was to provoke me into an argument about affirmative action. I sidestepped his daggers and responded calmly to his utterances, deflecting his comments, because I refused to play his game. When I got home that evening, I told my husband that I had been verbally violated, and I'd had to take it so as not to cause a scene. This faculty member was a white male professor who clearly felt entitled to treat me any way he chose. After that dinner I telepathically sent him a message to never, ever mess with me again. Perhaps he received the message, perhaps not, but I never had to deal with him again, thankfully. I could have engaged with him the way he wanted, and in all honesty, I could have defeated him, but at what cost? Where we were was neither the time nor the place for such a confrontation. These are the choices we sometimes face on a daily basis, choices that create ruptures in our sense of security when we have to *not* engage even though we have been deeply offended. These ruptures create cicatrices/scars in our minds, hearts, spirits, bodies. They are wounds with memory.

There are other aspects of academia that require a heightened awareness on our parts, aspects that deserve our scrutiny, aspects that should be called out for the harm they cause to our beings. Some of these include serving on countless committees to "talk about" diversity, equity, and inclusion; the nonrecognition of our extra service in mentoring students of color not only academically but personally; and ourselves sometimes falling prey to the notion of competition with each other. Also, just as we are observing the university, the university is also observing us. We need to manifest ourselves to the university, in no uncertain terms, that we know who we are and we will never let the university take that from us. This is our well-being.

VIII.

How we heal: *How is healing, protection, and support different from / the same as care work for students, for communities, for faculty?* The short answer is through solid, grounded, sincere communication. Through our *palabra,* our word(s), which reflect our worlds. Wor(l)d. Each of us comes from a world of our own, a world that contains circles upon circles composed of family, loved ones, friends, acquaintances. If we spun the wheel of difference, we would see that each of us comes from distinct positionalities. We identify according to a broad spectrum of attributes related to race, ethnicity, nationality, class, gender, religion/spirituality, culture(s), age/generation, urban/rural background, politics, ability/disability, health, and more. One of the factors that doesn't get mentioned as much as others is history (which Chandra Talpade Mohanty pointed out years ago). To me, perhaps history is the most important factor to remember when we are dealing with others. We sometimes know something about the history (or histories) of other communities, but we don't always know much about a person's history or how the complex factors that constitute an individual make her/him/them who they are. Here is where we must remember how crucial language is. Between a speaker and a listener, or a writer and a reader, words are what mediate in order to establish relation. Language, then, is crucial.

To live in community, we must know how to listen to each other. Deep listening. We must know how to see each other, be with each other, talk to each other. At the risk of sounding nostalgic, I want to acknowledge that at Davis, in the early years of our ethnic studies programs, the faculty from these programs were closer to each other. We met frequently and talked to each other. We stood in solidarity with each other. In recent times this energy has been missing. Perhaps in the earlier years, we knew what was at stake, we knew what we were all trying to build, and we respected our differences. And above all, we knew that we needed each other and that we would be there for each other. This sense of collectivity at this moment is fragile—in many ways, to be sure, due to the pandemic.

At the same time, all the ethnic studies programs can be tremendously powerful healing spaces. I am proud that at UC Davis, Native American Studies, Chicana/o Studies, Asian American Studies, and African and African American Studies chose to become independent, autonomous departments rather than allowing ourselves to be folded into an ethnic studies program or department. I have a mistrust of the ethnic studies paradigm because I see it as similar to the more recent offices of diversity, equity, and inclusion. Both seem to have an agenda of containing and controlling the growth of our disciplinary fields. At the same time, the scholars in ethnic studies programs, and those of us in autonomous departments, are working, via research and teaching, to break so many silences pertaining to the way our peoples have fared in U.S. society and how our peoples have responded, manifesting their own agency and ability to strategically talk back, fight back, and in every possible way subvert the intentions of any person or entity that would hold us back.

When all is said and done, I do believe that we can create community within academia, a community of like-minded, like-hearted individuals who are willing to work with each other to effect positive change in the institution, for our careers, for our lives, and for society. I reiterate. When you are in a community, you do not have to be best friends with everyone. It's OK to bond closely with some and not with others. The key is showing respect across differences. And if I may, to borrow from the Mapuche people of Chile (Nahuelpan 2009, 99), who regard tenderness as being paramount in their belief system, I do feel that in a community we can be tender with each other. Each person has a realm of privacy, their intimate spaces, that we do not know, or may not know, even if we are close to them. But when we think about this, we also have realms of privacy, intimate spaces that are ours, and ours alone. We must remember to reflect before we go into judgment. In our interactions with our colleagues, perhaps it would be good to remember Paulo Freire's (1970) pivotal question (paraphrased), "Is what you are doing serving the interests of oppression or of liberation?" Or as the Nimiipuu would say, from the perspective of our teachings, "Are you a light giver or a light taker? Are you a life giver or a life taker?"[5] For me, a true healing will be possible if we answer these questions by stepping back to see where we've come from and where we are now. *Una reflección.* A reflection that is both individual and collective. I know that in Chicanx studies, one overriding goal from more than fifty years ago was/is self-determination. In Native American studies, we emphasize sovereignty and autonomy. We must each know individually, profoundly, what self-determination/autonomy means, what it feels like, what it smells like, what it sounds like, what it tastes like, what it looks like. Here is the crux. To be able to envision collective autonomy (on

5. Phil Cash Cash, in conversation. I am a member of Luk'upsíimey / North Star Collective, which is a creative writing group of seven Nimiipuu / Nez Percé writers. We meet weekly to do language work, and particularly to integrate our language into our creative writing. This last passage regarding light givers and light takers references Phil Cash Cash's words from a conversation during one of our weekly meetings in late fall 2021.

campus, in community, in family, in circles of friends and colleagues), each of us has to practice a principled autonomy. Then we will join our light to the light of others, and our work and our lives will be illuminated, and this illumination will bring about our liberation, wherever we are, but certainly in academia, where so many of us have staked our lives. *Que así sea.*

References

Anzaldúa, Gloria. 2015. "Flights of the Imagination: Rereading/Rewriting Realities." In *Light in the Dark / Luz en lo oscuro: Rewriting Identity, Spirituality, Reality*, edited by AnaLouise Keating. Durham: Duke University Press.

Chihuailaf Nahuelpan, Elicura. 2009. *Message to Chileans*. Translated and with an introduction by Celso Cambiazo. Victoria, B.C.: Trafford.

Dumitrescu, Irina. 2019. "Ten Rules for Succeeding in Academia Through Upward Toxicity." *Times Higher Education*, November 21, 2019. https://www.timeshighereducation.com/opinion/ten-rules-succeeding-academia-through-upward-toxicity.

Freire, Paulo. 1970. *Pedagogy of the Oppressed*. Translated by Myra Bergman Ramos. New York: Seabury Press.

Lorde, Audre. 2007. "The Transformation of Silence into Language and Action." In *Sister Outsider: Essays and Speeches*, 40–44. Berkeley: Crossing Press.

Mohanty, Chandra Talpade. 1991. "Introduction." In *Cartographies of Struggle: Third World Women and the Politics of Feminism*, 1–47. Bloomington: Indiana University Press.

Womack, Craig. 2010. "Suspicioning: Imagining a Debate Between Those Who Get Confused, and Those Who Don't, When They Read Critical Responses to the Poems of Joy Harjo, or What's an Old-Timey Gay Boy like Me to Do?" *GLQ: A Journal of Lesbian and Gay Studies* 16 (1–2): 133–55.

Wood, Karenne. 2018. "The Poet I Wish I Was," In *New Poets of Native Nations*. Edited by Heid Erdrich.

CHAPTER 13

Hombres Latinos Saludables and Self-Care

HECTOR RIVERA-LOPEZ

In this essay, Hector Rivera-Lopez shares what he has learned about caregiving and self-care, as a Latinx clinical psychologist with more than fifty years of experience. This piece explores the following questions: Why do Latino men neglect self-care and place their health at risk? How do they learn to protect their own health? *"Aprendemos a cuidarnos a golpes"* (We learn to take care of ourselves through adversity) is a common response by Latino men when they are asked "How do you learn to take care of yourself?" but it is also a cry for help not heard by the same health institutions that are called on to help them.

"Eat your breakfast" (*Desayúnate*), "Keep yourself warm" (*Abrígate bien*), "Return home early" (*Regresa temprano a la casa*), "Stay out of trouble" (*No te metas en problemas*), "God bless you" (*Dios te bendiga*). Those were messages my mother gave me every time I left my home. These maternal "blessings" were intended to protect me and make sure that I stayed healthy and strong. Those "blessing messages" continued to resonate in my mind after many years.

How culture and families influence the quality of life of an individual and contribute to their success in life has been the focus of attention of some Latinx researchers, although the research on Latino men has been scarce and limited. This essay will explore Latino men's views on self-care and being healthy. I will give special attention to how men learn self-care within a gendered Puerto Rican and Latinx context.

But what is self-care? The New Oxford American Dictionary defines self-care as "the practice of taking action to preserve or improve one's own health." My remembrances and experiences growing up and the voices that contributed to shaping and influencing my attitude toward health are still on my mind. They are statements of love or "legacies of love" shaping my behavior in taking care of myself. When I reflected on how I learned self-care, two thoughts emerged: *mi mamá* (my mother) and *la calle* (the street). I became cognizant that self-care was mainly shaped by my mother's views (feminine view) and my street experiences (masculine view). It was between these two views or experiences that I forged a balance that provided cultural wisdom to face the challenges of everyday life, including my self-care.

I grew up in a culture where the essence of identity is grounded on the stories told. These stories influenced and shaped every aspect of my physical, psychological, and spiritual being. Listening to family stories, community stories, and political stories was central in my upbringing and socialization. Growing up and being raised as a Latino, I was told that I was responsible for the care of my family and those around me. I was expected to look after those who were weak and who needed my support and care. The only points of reference for performing this role or behavior were the stories of my family's male ancestors and the heroes from my culture. My performance was evaluated on my intensity and commitment to support and enact this role.

Many men grow up listening to narratives given by their caretakers but don't realize their power in defining their identity and personality. The message embedded in family narratives define who we are as men and how our lives are perceived and reacted to. These narratives are intended to help us cope with the challenges and realities unforeseen to us; in other words, they provide a legacy. These narratives are an important component of how our lives will be shaped.

Reflections on Self-Care

When I recall growing up in Puerto Rico and the experiences that shaped and influenced my view of life and self-care, my memories are rooted on my family of origin, especially my mother. I have vivid memories and images of my mother taking care of every single detail of the family and of my upbringing. I grew up in a middle-income Puerto Rican family; however, at the time, my options to pursue a college education were limited. The José Gautier Benítez High School, from which I graduated, had an educational counseling program that was very narrow in scope; I have no recollection of any instance in which the school provided information about pursuing a professional career after graduation. My educational options once I graduated in May 1967 were sparse. My choices were decided by the U.S. Army, *el servicio militar obligatorio* (the military draft). In 1967 the United States was fighting a nondeclared war in Vietnam (they called it a conflict); most of my neighborhood friends and peers were drafted and went to the army or to Vietnam to serve. My mother, who was a wise woman, was able to foresee my meager options and supported me in enrolling in college at the regional campus of the Catholic university. I was totally unaware that I could pursue a career and followed my mother's decision to continue my education. That was not the outcome for many of my friends, who were forced to join the army. My mother's devoted care contributed to the man that I have become today. As a statement of my gratitude to honor her, I kept her last name as part of my last name. Usually, in Latin American countries, we keep our two last names to honor our parents. When I migrated to the U.S. mainland on August 19, 1979, I decided to keep her last name: Lopez. This is my way to honor her sacrifice in raising me in Puerto Rico.

The other influence that taught me self-care was the street. In the streets, I learned how to survive and to cope with the inevitable unknown. From the wisdom of the streets, I learned to protect myself and be tough. Once I left the security of my family, I relied on the teachings of my family, to never give up and always trust myself. I carried with me my mother's wisdom and the streets' experience. Both together created a balance and informed my work with men as a clinical psychologist for nearly fifty years.

In the rest of this essay I will rely on client narratives to explore how Latino men think about self-care and their health belief model (Fowler et al. 2022), how they understand their health and the causes of illness, and how all these affect their lives and self-care practices. My analysis is also informed by observing and listening to Latino men's conversations about their experiences adjusting to and surviving the challenges of migrating to another country. Understanding how they learned about self-care during their migration and other situations is pivotal in promoting their physical, emotional, and spiritual well-being. How do men learn to take care of themselves? Who teaches them? What does it mean for a Latino male to say "I am taking care of myself"? How and under what circumstances are they willing to disclose issues about their well-being or health? These questions guide my analysis of client narratives.

All my professional life has been in my role as a psychologist within the context of the health care system and my own experience as a Latino growing up on the island of Puerto Rico. My interest in men's health stems from my dad. My dad was a wonderful and responsible man who woke up every morning around three o'clock to go to work. The weather was never an impediment to him in pursuing his obligations; neither were illnesses. Every morning I heard him waking up and getting ready to face the challenges of the incoming day. He worked for a soda company, driving a truck and delivering the product to local businesses in the community. He never complained about the hard work, despite the stress and job demands. I remember hearing the reasons behind his commitment to work for a national company that never honored or appreciated his work, except for a little gold medal given to all employees who never missed a day of labor. I remember attending the annual company party where employees were recognized for their loyalty

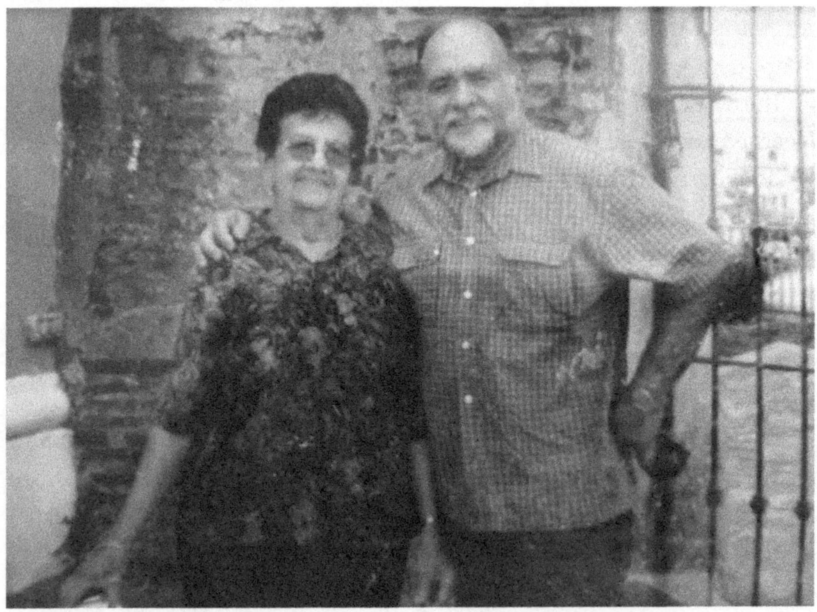

FIGURE 13.1 Me and my mom after Dad died of cancer.

and commitment to the company and were given a little pin with a monetary bonus. During his thirty-plus years working for this company, he collected many of those little pins. He was always proud of his impeccable commitment to his job. When I asked him "Have you ever gotten sick enough to miss a day of work?" he responded with a very serious tone: "Who will bring food to the table of our family?" His loyalty to the values with which he grew up (pride in his job performance and self-respect for himself) and his comments still resonate with me. His loyalty to the company and what it represented for him were more powerful than his commitment to his self-care. His commitment was influenced by his obligations to his family, a central tenet for Latino men. This story is the story of my father, who died less than two years after his retirement. He devoted over thirty years to his company and never held any other job during his life. He was sixty-eight years old when he died from a preventable cancer. When he sought medical help, it was too late. It was my mother who took him to all his medical appointments and provided care. The story of my father exemplifies those of many Latino men.

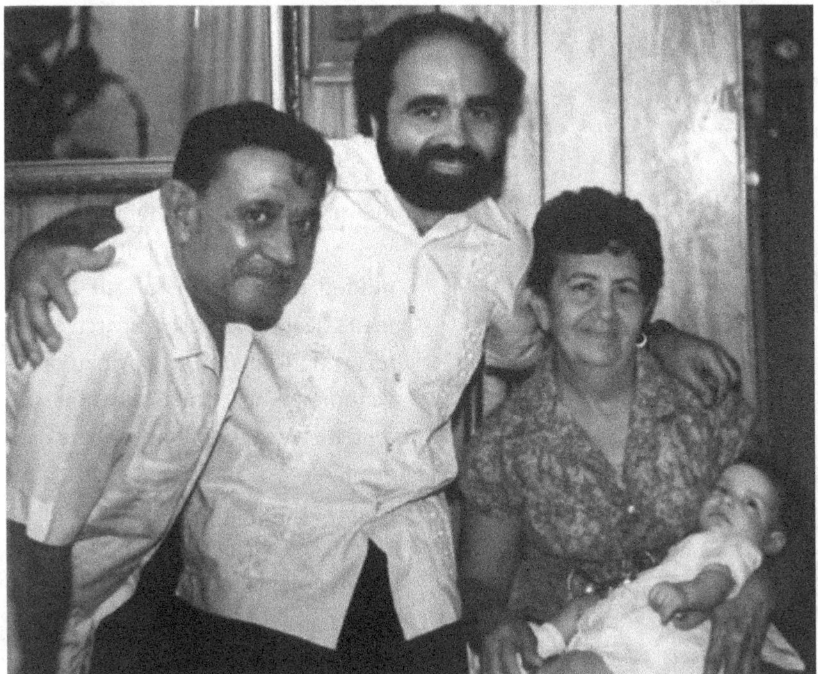

FIGURE 13.2 Mom, Dad, and me, age thirty-two, with my young niece.

Latino Men and Self-Care

My mother informed my knowledge and practice of self-care through her words and actions; my father modeled what men should not do—sacrifice their health to fulfill a cultural mandate. As stated previously, there is limited research regarding how Latino men learn and practice self-care. Most of the health information available is focused on secondary or tertiary health prevention; that is, the prevalence and incidence of disease among Latinxs (see CDC 2022). Research interventions focusing on preventing illness (primary prevention) is practically nonexistent. Most of the data available on Latinx physical health derives from consultations with physicians when a man feels ill or has been diagnosed with a disease. In brief medical visits, the focus is on diagnosing or managing the illness, not on learning about the patients' health beliefs or self-care practices. For patients with chronic illnesses, such as hypertension, cardiovascular disease, or diabetes, which are prevalent among Latinos, understanding self-care practices is critical to managing disease. However, these conversations tend to occur when illness has progressed, not in primary prevention efforts.

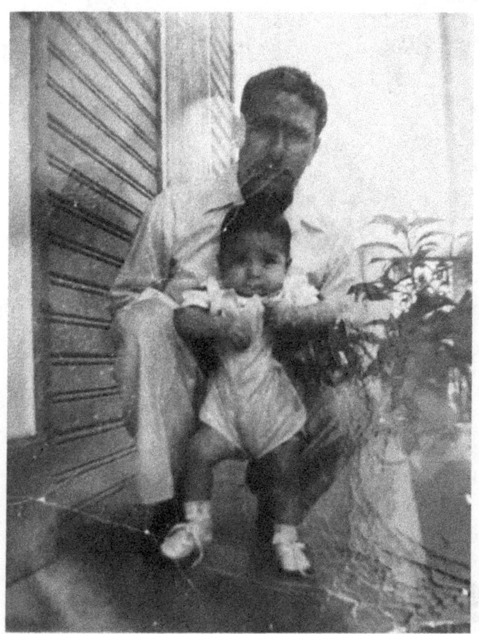

FIGURE 13.3 Me, age one, and Dad.

This lack of information represents a challenge for helping professionals because primary measures or strategies to support Latino men's health are practically nonexistent. Also, the lack of data has contributed to misguided assumptions about Latino men's health. Because research or interventions focusing on primary prevention are also practically nonexistent, this means that most of the data available on this population come from Latino men who have gone to visit their available health practitioner when sick or when they have a disease. This lack of data creates and promotes misguided assumptions about Latinx health attitudes, which can affect the doctor-patient relationship and the quality of health care received. For example, when I was in conversation with a friend of mine, he shared an experience that he'd had in a recent visit to his cardiologist. Before he met the doctor, the nurse took his blood pressure (BP), with a reading of 170/90. The doctor immediately told him that his BP was too high; thus, he was going to increase his BP medication without considering one possible reason for the reading, what is referred to as the white-coat syndrome—that is, visiting the doctor often elevates the BP of patients. When my friend told the doctor that every day he measures his BP and the range is consistently between 126/72 and 137/76, the doctor responded, "Your machine doesn't work." My friend decided to go against his doctor's advice to increase his BP medication. The doctor responded, "You are an intelligent man; do what you want. But I am going to document the BP reading in your medical file."

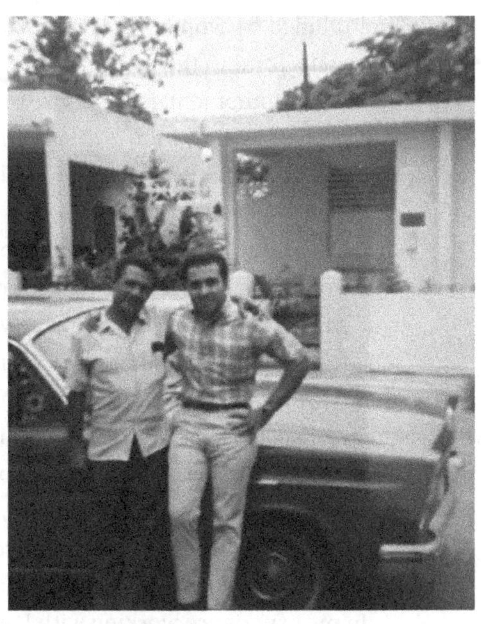

FIGURE 13.4 Dad and me, age sixteen.

Women as Facilitators of Care

There is a saying in Spanish, "*Detrás del éxito de un hombre hay siempre una mujer*" (Behind the success of a man there is always a woman). This saying reflects an irrefutable truth among many Latinx cultures, and many men abide by this unwritten rule. Writing this chapter, I rephrase the saying as "*Detrás de la salud de un hombre siempre existe una mujer*" (Behind a man's health there is always a woman).

How do most Latinos take care of themselves? Early in their childhoods, Latinos are raised to take care of others, and their needs are usually taken care of by females. Most of the time the mother (or a maternal figure such as a grandmother) is the caregiver of men. If this "arrangement" is honored or implemented, most males are comfortable with their needs being anticipated and fulfilled by women. It is important to mention that Latinos in general are totally loyal to the mother figure in allowing them to take care of themselves. Any other female (wives, sisters, cousins, and female friends) often is approached with caution and sometimes mistrust. Usually men don't want to "own" to anybody any behaviors that reveal that they are not self-reliant or dependable enough.

Demonstrating that they are capable of and able to take care of others and themselves is a matter of pride and respect. Within the context of a patriarchal culture where women are perceived as caregivers, women often perform a delicate dance of taking care of men, including their health (thus fulfilling their own mandate), without making it appear that the man depends on them for such needs to preserve his dignity, lest he appear or feel weak or dependent. The main role that women play in supporting, teaching, and caring for others physically, psychologically, and spiritually is paramount in Latinx cultures. Women's role on teaching self-care is a major point of reference in the way men perceive, understand, and apply this teaching to themselves.

In my experience working with Latino heterosexual immigrant men, they often have little information about their health and refer health questions to their spouses. However, it is important to note that Latinos are also caregivers of women, albeit in a traditional way, by often being the primary financial provider and taking care of instrumental gender-based chores like doing yardwork, taking care of garbage, et cetera. This is central to the gender role of Latino men (see Flores at al. 2020). Taking care of men's health often takes the form enacted by my mother, through *consejos* (advice) and insisting men seek health care when ill, as was the case with my father and many men with whom I have worked.

Working with Latino Men in Groups

For the last forty years, one of my areas of interest as a community clinical psychologist has focused on men's health and how men take care of themselves. Since 2018 I have been conducting a weekly Latino men's group sponsored by a local school district in the eastern region of Contra Costa County in California. It is not a psychotherapy group but a psychoeducational support group with the principal goal of creating a safe environment to facilitate the men's discussion of the concerns and worries encountered in their daily lives. The group consists of eleven immigrant Latino men from different countries, but mainly from Mexico. Their ages range from thirty years old to seventy-one; the mean age is forty-five.

All the men in the group joined voluntarily and were referred by their wives or other relatives. An interesting fact was that half the men attending the group were survivors of catastrophic diseases, such as cardiovascular disease, diabetes, stroke, and spinal cord injuries. All the men were married and had children, and most were at the peak of their work productivity. Many of them were on medical leave (unable to work because of illness or injury) or retired because of health problems. When they were asked why they came to the group, the consensus was that it was because their wives, mothers, or close relatives thought they could benefit from it.

How can a counselor or group leader conduct a group of Latino men facing the above health problems with their attendant psychological and social challenges? To address this question, it is important to understand the cultural values inherent in the concept of self-care. There is not a clear consensus about what self-care means for Latino men. For Latino men, being healthy implies a sense of independence from others. *"El hombre verdadero no depende de otros para resolver los problemas"* (A real man doesn't rely on others to face his personal problems). All members of the groups I have facilitated collectively shared this statement, which applies not only to social issues but to health problems as well. Latino men are immensely proud of how they care for their families, children, and others in their extended family or support system, for example, compadres, friends, neighbors, and even strangers.

In my early professional days working as a psychologist in the community mental health system of Puerto Rico, I had an experience that I vividly remember. A thirty-year-old woman was scheduled to have a cesarean procedure in the hospital adjacent to the community mental health center. She developed a severe depression with catatonic features because of her fears of having the surgery. She was hospitalized in our mental health program to address her depressive symptoms and to help her prepare for the cesarean. When she was closer to delivering her baby, she was still not ready to embrace the surgical procedure, and the doctors were worried about the outcome. The situation became more difficult and complex because her blood type was O negative, a type not common among the Puerto Rican population. Her husband was informed about the situation and was given the task of finding people willing to donate blood that matched his wife's blood type, an endeavor that he immediately initiated. I remember the morning that he brought six males to do the testing for the blood type match.

None of them stayed to do the testing, and all left the hospital premises, creating a major health crisis because the woman was already in the process to have the cesarean procedure. Luckily for the hospital and the patient, my blood type matched hers, and I donated the blood. This case is a vivid example that illustrates the value many Latino men place on supporting others in need but also demonstrates the limited knowledge many Latino men have about their own bodies and the importance of taking care of themselves. For example, the potential blood donors the patient's husband brought to the hospital early in the morning were under the influence of alcohol (they were not drunk but had been actively drinking the night before), and none of them was aware that being under the influence disqualified them as blood donors. Although they arrived to the hospital to donate blood, the fact that alcohol was evident in their bodies (on their breath) eliminated them as blood donors.

Latino Health Narratives

In the traditional Latinx context, a man who complains about his health is perceived as weak or not strong. Many of the men I have worked with had very limited understanding about how their bodies work. Thus, in our groups, the topic of self-care is approached with caution and hesitation. For many Latino men, help is sought due to illness or only when the body no longer tolerates pain. In most cases it is the wife or partner who will advocate and "force" the men to seek help.

The lives of many Latino men are in crisis, and so is their health. When the members of the group were asked "How do you learn about self-care?" their typical response was "I learn *a golpes*" (the hard way). The men meant that when they face a health crisis and realize that they are not prepared to respond to it, they feel worried and desperate. Then they are more likely to seek help. Many of the men in the groups I lead are willing to listen and learn but lack the necessary skills/strategies to practice self-care. Often these men have no place to talk about the impact of their health condition and the burden it places on them or on their loved ones. Symptoms of anxiety and depression, including poor sleep, irritability, lack of interest in daily activity, fatigue, low libido, and becoming easily annoyed by minor details of daily life, are manifestations of their lack of more adaptive responses to illness. When stoicism and reliance on *aguantarse* no longer function as ways of coping, the men do not know what to do. Emotional isolation and refusal to understand what is happening or explain their situation to others (family members or friends) indicate their struggle to share their intimate thoughts about what they are experiencing. For many of these men, their socialization process emphasized performance of their gender role without complaint (see Flores et al. 2020).

Martin is a forty-seven-year-old male.[6] He was referred to the group by his wife, who became aware of the group Hombres Creando Lazos de Comunidad. He joined the group when a series of events in his life contributed to symptoms of depression and anxiety. He was diagnosed with severe depression and was under medical care and medication. He reported, "I can't shake out feelings of emptiness and depression" and "My life no longer has meaning." He shared with the group that he was a burden to his immediate family and other relatives and didn't know what to do despite seeing his primary physician in a local HMO. Finding community with other Latino men in the group helped break his isolation and recover most of his energy and passion for life. After a few group meetings, he stated "My life has a meaning again." This participant has been in the group for more than seven months and is always on time to the meetings.

Years ago, I facilitated a men's group, Compadres Sin Fronteras, in the city of Concord, California. This group lasted more than thirteen years. It was a support group with the main goal of co-creating a safe space for men to discuss in the company of other men the challenges and daily problems they faced. The group provided participants with a space to talk about their concerns and struggles. One experience related to my work with that group was related to prostate health. I was invited by a local HMO to extend an invitation to Compadres Sin Fronteras to attend a regional men's health fair. At that time, I was a board member for the American Cancer Society and chose as my contribution to the society the education of Latino men about prostate health issues. To my surprise, few men knew what a prostate was or about the health issues related to it. I provided them health information from the American Cancer Society and explained to them what constituted a prostate

---

6. Informed consent was obtained to use the narratives included in this paper. Pseudonyms have been used.

examination. Many of the men reacted with anxiety and nervousness, which in Latinx cultures may translate into jokes and laughter. At the end of the presentation, many of them refused to have their prostate examined. Some of the men were afraid of having blood drawn, and others (the majority) rejected the idea of a physician performing a digital rectal examination. Lack of information about their bodies, the stigma associated with a digital rectal examination, and concerns about their masculinity were putting these men's lives at risk. This is of great concern, given the high rates of prostate cancer among Latino men. Prostate cancer is the most commonly diagnosed cancer among Latino men in the United States, comprising more than one in five of all new cancer diagnoses and contributing more than seventeen thousand new diagnoses and two thousand deaths annually (GLOBOCAN 2012).

I have found that many men hold inside them oppressive narratives that never were disclosed and have produced in them high levels of stress. Often these men use metaphors to describe their life situations because they cannot speak directly about their wounding. For example, I was leading a Latino men's support group presentation on how to cope with anxiety and stress during the COVID-19 pandemic when Daniel, one of the participants, shared with the group that he was facing a stressful situation with his immediate supervisor and was considering quitting his job, which he had held for over ten years. He described the female supervisor's behavior as characterized by "*sangre pesada*" / "*sangre ligera*" (heavy blood / soft blood). This metaphor symbolized his impotence in coping with the stress the supervisor's inflexible attitude caused him. "Heavy blood" refers to her inflexible attitude and "soft blood" to her flexibility toward him. Sharing his work situation led him to share with other group participants a narrative about his family of origin that has influenced and burdened his relationship with females. His mother had migrated to the USA with his younger sister, leaving him behind, under the care of his maternal grandmother. He was five years old then and felt betrayed and abandoned. Even though his mother's main reason for migration was to improve the family financial situation, Daniel felt rejected and resentful toward her. This case illustrates how narratives men secretly hold and that they keep inside can adversely affect their health and well-being as well as their relationships with others.

The anger and stress contained in old memories may foster impotence and frustration, often driving men to cope by means of alcohol consumption. Alcohol misuse contributes to illness and is quite prevalent among Latino men (Carrillo and Zarza 2008). Drinking as a strategy to cope with stress is commonly learned in the streets. Even though Daniel had graduated from a prestigious college in the United States, he did not know how to care for himself.

Juan, a Latino male who migrated to the USA at the young age of twenty-one, also repressed a painful narrative. In the United States he began to work in a meatpacking company. By the age of twenty-seven he was married, had two daughters, and was a stroke survivor. When he joined the group, he was thirty years old and had been referred by his wife, who had "forced" him to attend the group; otherwise, she would leave him and return to her family of origin. Juan was incredibly angry and resentful about his health condition and how the illness was affecting his marital life and family. When other men began to share their health struggles and impediments, Juan began to open up and became an active participant. As he shared his painful migration narrative, he began to see the connection between his story and his illness.

One factor each participant had in common was their limited knowledge about how their bodies function and work. Most of them were driven to perform according to the cultural scripts imposed on them and were not assuming an active role in taking care of themselves. An outcome the group offered them was to advocate and educate other Latino men about the importance of playing an active role in taking care of themselves. For those participants (half the group) who were survivors of a catastrophic illness, becoming aware that they were prisoners of their own bodies (physically) and beginning to understand the power of sharing narratives that oppressed them was an act of liberation that created possibilities. Developing healthy lifestyles was a new experience to free their mind and spirit to seek new *fronteras* (frontiers).

Conclusions

The narratives of Latino men foreground several themes, including their lack of knowledge about their bodies, the factors affecting their health, the importance of self-care, their reliance on women to monitor and safeguard their health, and the danger of sacrificing their bodies to fulfill a cultural mandate. As stated, Latino men are immensely proud of caring for their families and others but fall short in taking care of themselves. Drawing on my many years of working with men, in this section I offer strategies for health organizations to address this situation. Influencing Latino men's existing beliefs about self-care and creating alternatives to improve their self-care is of utmost importance for future generations.

1. Develop strategies to teach their members self-care, especially Latino men.
2. Focus on how to understand and deliver services to meet the health needs of Latino men by developing culturally based strategies that promote and maintain well-being.
3. Increase Latinx staff, including health care providers and health educators who understand the cultural values and health beliefs of diverse Latinx patients and the cultural scripts that affect men's health.
4. Train staff to learn, understand, and respect the cultural value system that influences and informs Latinx health beliefs.
5. Understand that respect and honor are important values held by Latino men and are to be acknowledged.
6. Develop strategies to address Latinx needs embedded in a collaborative approach to bring them as co-authors of the interventions implemented.

References

Carrillo, C., and M. J. Zarza. 2008. "Fire and Firewater: A Co-Occurring Clinical Treatment Model for Domestic Violence, Substance Abuse, and Trauma." In *Family Violence and Men of Color*, edited by J. Tello and R. Carrillo, 61–84. 2nd edition. New York: Springer.

CDC (Centers for Disease Control and Prevention). 2022. "Health of Hispanic or Latino Population." CDC/National Center for Health Statistics, October 19, 2022. https://www.cdc.gov/nchs/fastats/hispanic-health.htm.

Flores, Y., L. Brazil-Cruz, H. Rivera-Lopez, R. Manzo, M. Sianez, and Erika Cervantes Pacheco. 2020. "Aquí en confianza (Here in Confidence): Narratives of Migration, Mental Health, and Family Reunification of Mexican Immigrant Men in the California Central Valley." In *Community-Based Participatory Research: Testimonios from Chicana/o Studies*, edited by Natalia Deeb-Sossa, 153–78. Tucson: University of Arizona Press.

Fowler, A. L., M. E. Mann, F. J. Martinez, H.-W. Yeh, and J. D. Cowden. 2022. "Cultural Health Beliefs and Practices Among Hispanic Parents." *Clinical Pediatrics* 61 (1): 56–65. https://doi.org/10.1177/00099228211059666.

GLOBOCAN 2012. 2012. Cancer Incidence and Mortality Worldwide (database), version 1.0. International Agency for Research on Cancer.

Stern, M. C. 2020. "Prostate Cancer in US Latinos: What Have We Learned and Where Should We Focus Our Attention." In *Advancing the Science of Cancer in Latinos*, edited by A. G. Ramirez and E. J. Trapido, 57–67. Cham, Switzerland: Springer. https://www.ncbi.nlm.nih.gov/books/NBK573249/.

PART III

Reflection

Caregiver Bill of Rights

The collaborators to this volume co-created this Caregiver Bill of Rights. This list was modified from Jo Horne's Caregiving: Helping an Aging Loved One. *We invite the reader to create their own statement of rights using this list. Read the list to yourself every day.*

• • •

I have the right to the following:

to acknowledge that caretaking is deeply rooted in patriarchal, homophobic, and transphobic models of caretaking in marriage, childbearing/childrearing, and family units;

to work to dismantle patriarchy, homophobia, and transphobia when I caretake;

to expect that my positionality and identities are respected;

to create a culturally competent health care system, oriented and informed by social justice, that recognizes and acts on social disparities and differences;

to develop and nurture queer, muxerista, intersectional communities that will help teach those who care for others;

to practice radical feminist self-love, self-care, and collective love and care;

to be rooted in a loving, healing, and compassionate practice;

to identify the impact of mental and spiritual illness and focus on healing to prevent this illness;

to be a better caretaker of myself and others;

to expect that caregiving responsibilities are not placed on my shoulders alone;

to expect that others will care for me in healthy ways as I care for them and others;

to tell my story, and to have it listened to and acted on;

to receive outreach from others and to advocate for my care recipient and myself;

to celebrate my own individual and community forms of caregiving;

to receive consideration, appreciation, and acceptance for all I do for care recipient, family, friends, community, and society at large;

to take care of myself so I may retain the capacity to care for my care recipient and myself;

to seek help from others, as I recognize the limits of my own endurance and strength;

to resist conscious or unconscious attempts by my care recipient to rely on guilt, anger, or depression;

to receive consideration, affection, forgiveness, and acceptance from care recipients when I offer them in return;

to take pride in what I am accomplishing and applaud the courage it has taken me to meet the needs of my care recipient;

to prioritize myself and maintain facets of my own life that do not always include the person I care for, just as I would if they were healthy;

to protect my individuality and my right to make a life for myself that will sustain me in the time when my care recipient no longer needs my full-time help;

to expect and demand that as new strides are made in finding resources to aid physically and mentally impaired older persons in our country, similar strides will be made toward aiding and supporting caregivers;

to occasionally express anger and other difficult feelings regarding the caregiving situation I am in and to experience a peaceful and calm atmosphere while giving care;

to secure systemic support from institutions and the government to take care of others;

to partake of a society that values, support, and nurtures caring;

to connect with those who care for others and care within community;

to live in a society that values caring for all and that encourages all to be caregivers of our children, youth, and elders; and

to be treated with, and to treat myself with, dignity and respect, and to give thanks for being alive and for being given the opportunity to caretake another day.

Reference

Horne, Jo. 1985. *Caregiving: Helping an Aging Loved One*. Washington, D.C.: American Association of Retired Persons.

Reflection

A Call to Action

ANGIE CHABRAM, NATALIA DEEB-SOSSA, AND YVETTE G. FLORES

We conclude this volume with an invitation to readers to document their caregiving and healing stories. It is imperative that we develop archives that will provide lessons of advocacy, relationality, and community agency and interpretation if we are to gain an understanding of the breadth and depth of Latina/o/x care experiences in the global period and beyond. From our standpoint these archives cover a wide range of geographical, social, and creative forms of expression that are plentiful in everyday life, although not always recognized.

These archives are also an extension of community knowledge making; they contain valuable lessons, *consejos*, and insights that cannot be found in mainstream renditions of caregiving. They inscribe caregiving in meaningful community contexts that shape health and healing processes. They draw our attention to all the unforeseen places where instances of care work can be found. They identify forms of care work that are not usually associated with this practice within society. They extend care to social processes such as immigration, education, and nutrition. They encapsulate the new ethnicities and *latinidades* of our time; they unite the Americas with a larger worldwide village of care workers and receivers. They provide hope that something can be done even when it appears that this is not the case. They are replete with caregiver *soldaderas* who extend human rights to the area of social care and in so doing deprivatize one of the world's oldest professions. They shine a light on the essential care provided by women who are often characterized as carers without attention to their contributions or the ways in which they self-consciously assume this work or modify gender relations. Most important, they rewrite themselves into the caregiver narrative by insisting that they not only provide but also receive care and that their labor also includes self-care. These *testimonios* represent multigenerational narratives of women and one man who engage in diverse forms of employment in addition to care work, contrary to the stereotype of Latinas who are homemakers and mostly do care work. Most of the contributors come from working-class backgrounds, are first-generation college students, and have made a commitment to using their academic work and writings to advocate and elevate their communities.

These testimonios also embody and highlight the importance of the disability justice framework, which understands that all bodies are unique and essential; all bodies care, work, and have strengths and needs that must be met. All *testimonialistas* are, in their own way, doing disability justice work. When doing disability justice work, it becomes impossible not to look at disability, not examine how colonialism created it, and not see that disability is evident in Black and brown, queer and trans communities. The message and vision of the volume is liberation that understands that the government will not care for our loved ones because it was created to erase us (Piepzna-Samarasinha 2018, 182). The testimonialistas also ask, If we do not have family or social networks rooted in activism and solidarity, who is going to be there for me?

This volume is mixed genre and includes pieces of personal testimony and poetry, meditations, and a mix of tools that worked for the authors. We hope you can learn from the stories shared and care for each other while caring for yourself. Most important, these testimonios and archives often answer the following questions:

- What happens when there is no doctor or nurse around?
- Who is at the helm of care?
- Who delivers vital forms of care that are necessary for survival?
- Who can be counted on when doctors don't understand, when there is no health care, or when the need surpasses the doctor's visit?
- Who can serve as interpreter, not only of language but of the health beliefs and cultural values that create nuance in the experience of illness and caregiving and receiving?

- Who will hold our memories and speak to our needs when aging, dementia, or cognitive decline takes away our ability to advocate for ourselves?
- Who will look after our elderly family members who can't afford to live independently?

Representational archives provide a presence to community members at the margins of society who are in need of two-way dialogues and a circulation of critical forms of knowledge and practice. For this reason, we urge our readers to reenter the field of narrative work with an open mind and a commitment to gathering and producing caregiver narratives that surround every significant human ailment, including the isms we are all too familiar with: racism, classism, sexism, ageism, fatphobia, ignorance, and heterosexism.

As we reflect on our journey of caregiving, we foreground the ways in which *cultura*, gender, intergenerational histories, and traumas manifest in our care practices. Our testimonios present in unique ways how we can resist health care models that dehumanize, marginalize, and disregard personal agency, that prioritize medical expertise over a person's knowledge of their body. The authors challenge the patriarchal order and contest and transform gendered scripts that idealize *familia* and are rooted in precarious *familismo*—that is, a family-centeredness that privileges cisgender straight men and overburdens women and queer Latinxs who have no children of their own. In the caregiving context, precarious familismo mandates caring for family members through the sacrifice of some. These testimonios also offer self and community advocacy and model community care and self-care. They ask the questions, Who is going to show up? How do we transcend the difficulty of asking for help when we have been brainwashed by bootstrap individualism?

The authors also highlight the resiliency of the human spirit, manifested in the narratives of our contributors, like in the cases of ire'ne lara silva and Maria R. Palacios. Enriqueta Valdez-Curiel utilizes the cultural capital her medical degree affords her and her transnational experience as a child of immigrants to navigate her mother's care in Mexico and the United States. Recognizing the privilege her education affords her, she lovingly provides care for her mother while advocating for quality health care that ultimately saves her mother's life. Similarly, Angie Chabram, availing herself of her mother's teachings of familial co-caregiving and employing her cultural capital as a University of California professor, caregives for her mother, with support of her sister and brothers. Natalia Deeb-Sossa witnesses her partner's struggle with the medical establishment and moves beyond a caregiver role of providing emotional support to become his advocate, challenging the medical system and fighting for appropriate care while navigating her own health struggles. Both of these testimonios underscore the importance of self-care and the toll caregiving can take on the health and emotional well-being of family caregivers.

In each of the testimonios, we see the authors' contestation of gendered cultural scripts and a contestation of precarious familismo. Josie Méndez-Negrete must balance her love for her son and her activism for him to obtain the care he needs with her career and other family responsibilities. Her testimonio and Anita Tijerina Revilla's visibilize the impact of mental illness on the family and the ways in which caregivers must step up and take over decisions and choices for the affected individual to protect them. Anita Tijerina Revilla's testimonio demonstrates a Muxerista feminist praxis of care as she becomes her niece and nephew's guardian and mobilizes a community and social system to raise the children into well-functioning adults while advocating for her sister, who is not receiving the care she needs.

Anita Tijerina Tijerina Revilla poignantly describes the ravages of addiction and mental health and the trauma it causes across generations, as well as the limitations of a capitalist health care system. Her testimonio also invites us to reflect on traditional kinship roles and the importance of community, whether we are providing care for our children; raising our grandchildren, as in yvonne hurtado allen's case; or caring for an in-law, as in Maria Soltandenko's case. Gender-based expectations concerning who should provide care are contested in each of these testimonios.

Our focus was to include caregiving practices often ignored in narratives of care. Natalia Deeb-Sossa and Mónica Torreiro-Casal offer us insights into their commitment to support minoritized students and create a space of belonging for those who are often disenfranchised in academic settings. This is an added tax, often invisible to the larger institution, on being a Chicana faculty member who not only instructs and mentors but also protests. These faculty members' caregiving of students is an act of love, resistance, and empowerment. Inés Hernández-Ávila's testimonio denounces the racist, capitalist academic systems that are designed to exclude working-class, minoritized women and people of color from its student ranks and that assault the bodies, psyches, and souls of faculty of color. Giving voice to the macro- and microaggressions women of color who are academics experience, Inés Hernández-Ávila challenges us all to interrogate our internalized self-deprecation that can and often does lead women of color to turn against other women of color. Inés Hernández-Ávila also provides valuable insights on self-care and how to survive the toxicity of academic spaces.

The caregiving narratives also include those by professional caregivers who transcend their training. The testimonios foreground the ways in which professional care providers Hector Rivera-Lopez and Yvette G. Flores resist Western models of "appropriate" psychotherapy and rely on a culturally rooted ethics of care (Flores et al. 2009) that humanizes care and breaks down the power imbalance inherent in psychologist-client relationships. Hector Rivera-Lopez's testimonio offers a nuanced view of men's reliance on women for their own self-care and their neglect of their own health as they attempt to fulfill their masculine role of provider, which results in early death and disability. His testimonio highlights the ways in which men learn to care for themselves, at home and on the streets, and how through loving therapeutic encounters, he helps the men understand the burden of their masculinity, their entitlement to health, and their unconscious expectations that the women in their lives should be in charge of their health and well-being. Both Yvette G. Flores and Hector Rivera-Lopez underscore the importance of self-care while caring for others in their professional roles.

We see the authors' narratives as efforts to break intergenerational patterns of exclusion, trauma, invisibility, pain, and silence. Whether struggling with the ravages of diabetes, cancer, dementia, disability, addiction, or historical trauma, the contributors shed light on how their intersectional identities—working-class origins, family histories, and current positionalities as academics, poets, activist scholars—provide resilience and a road map to navigate complex systems and challenging situations.

We then invite our readers to share their testimonios or archives of caregiving with friends, family, and other caregivers through *pláticas* (heart-to-heart conversations) in which they can share the courage it takes to be a communal and familial caregiver. Our hope is that this volume will encourage others to share their knowledge about caregiving to build solidarity and respond to and resist structures of oppression that promote invisibility and exclusion in the medical-industrial complex.

Finally, we hope that in *Testimonios of Care: Feminist Latina/x and Chicana/x Perspectives on Caregiving Praxis* we have given voice to those who often are voiceless in histories of caregiving and that diverse caregivers see themselves reflected, valued, and thus honored completely: body-mind-spirit (Lara 2002; Facio and Lara 2014). The testimonios of caregiving highlight a loving relationship that binds the caregiver to their loved one through the attesting of their health, illness, and pain. The testimonios underscore how care receivers also reciprocate the care received in their own unique ways.

References

Facio, Elisa, and Lara, Irene, eds. 2014. *Fleshing the Spirit: Spirituality and Activism in Chicana, Latina, and Indigenous Women's Lives*. Tucson: University of Arizona Press.

Flores, Yvette G., Ladson Hinton, Judith C. Baker, Carol E. Franz, and Alexandra Velasquez. 2009. "Beyond Familism: Ethics of Care of Latina Caregivers of Elderly Parents with Dementia." *Health Care for Women International* 30 (12): 1055–72.

Lara, Irene. 2002. "Healing Sueños for Academia." In *This Bridge We Call Home: Radical Visions for Transformations*, edited by Gloria E. Anzaldúa and AnaLouise Keating, 433–38. New York: Routledge.

Piepzna-Samarasinha, L. L. 2018. *Care Work: Dreaming Disability Justice*. Vancouver: Arsenal Pulp Press.

Contributors

yvonne hurtado allen earned an undergraduate degree in sociology from Woodland Community College and a master's degree in regional and community development and a PhD in education from the University of California, Davis, as an older nontraditional student. yvonne's experiential knowledge, gained through childhood poverty, a lifetime of low-income jobs, and living in low-income neighborhoods, has given her a unique perspective with which to connect with many of her students and their experiences and realities. yvonne has experienced many of the same issues as the students she now instructs and is able to draw on her life experiences as well as her education to guide and mentor with insight and awareness. Dr. hurtado allen is currently a lecturer at University of California, Davis, in the Department of Chicana/o Studies and teaches at a local community college. She has an article and a book chapter under review and is working on an article based on her dissertation.

Angie Chabram is professor emerita at the University of California, Davis. Her publications span the fields of Chicana/o cultural studies, literary criticism, feminism, narrative health, and identity. She is the youngest daughter of Angie G. Chabram, single parent of four.

Natalia Deeb-Sossa is a professor in Chicana/o Studies at the University of California, Davis, who has more than sixteen years teaching in public higher education. Dr. Deeb-Sossa is active in the movement for ethnic studies, being the co-chair of the University of California Ethnic Studies Council and in the Davis Joint Unified School District Ethnic Studies Advisory Committee. Her latest co-edited book, *Latinx Belonging: Community Building and Resilience in the United States* (2022), with Dr. Jennifer Bickham Mendez (University of

Arizona Press), positions Latinxs' struggles for recognition and inclusion as squarely located within intersecting power structures of gender, race, sexuality, and class and as shaped by state-level and transnational forces such as U.S. immigration policies and histories of colonialism.

Yvette G. Flores obtained a doctoral degree in clinical psychology at the University of California, Berkeley, in 1982. She has done postdoctoral work in health psychology. Her research focus includes substance abuse treatment outcome, women's mental health, intimate partner violence, and the mental health of immigrant men. A professor of psychology in Chicana/o Studies at the University of California, Davis, for the past thirty-three years, Dr. Flores was co-investigator of a National Science Foundation Institutional Transformation grant to increase the numbers of Latinas with careers in science, technology, engineering, mathematics, and medicine. Her publications reflect her life's work of bridging community-clinical psychology and Chicanx/Latinx studies, as she foregrounds gender, ethnicity, and sexualities in her clinical, teaching, and research practice. Her book *Chicana and Chicano Mental Health: Alma, Mente y Corazón* was published by the University of Arizona Press in 2013, while the first edition of *Psychological Perspectives on Chicanx and Latinx Families* was published by Cognella Academic Publishing in 2014. Sentia Publishing published her e-book on Latinx children and adolescents in 2016. Her co-authored book *Cultura y Corazón: A Decolonial Methodology for Community Engaged Research* was published in 2020 by University of Arizona Press. She is the co-author with Prof. Mónica Torreiro-Casal of two books: *Chicanx and Latinx Psychology: A Decolonial Approach* (Great River Learning, 2022) and *Psychological Perspectives on Chicanx and Latinx Families* (Cognella, 2021).

Dr. Flores is a national and international consultant on cultural humility; prevention and treatment of trauma; and gender, migration, and mental health. Dr. Flores was recently promoted to distinguished professor at the University of California, Davis.

Inés Hernández-Ávila (Nimiipuu / Nez Percé and Tejana) is professor of Native American Studies at the University of California, Davis, and one of the six founders of the Native American and Indigenous Studies Association. Her research focuses on the interrelationships between autonomy, spirit, ways of knowing and being, the arts, and social justice through the study of Native American / Indigenous poetry, United States / Mexico, with a particular focus on Chiapas, and through her work on Indigenous religious traditions of the Americas. She is a poet, translator, visual artist, and member of Luk'upsíimey / North Star Collective, a group of Nimiipuu creative writers and language workers. In August 2022 she traveled with members of Luk'upsíimey to Chiapas, Mexico, to meet with Mayan counterparts. She collaborated with the Library of Congress to produce the PALABRA Indigenous Voices Project (https://guides.loc.gov/palabra-archive/indigenous-voices); the site has recordings by twelve Mayan writers of Chiapas, with their photos and biographies. She holds a Distinguished Teaching Award from the UC Davis Academic Senate. In April 2017 she received the Frank Bonilla Public Intellectual Award from the Latino Studies section of the Latin American Studies Association.

ire'ne lara silva is the author of four poetry collections, *furia, Blood Sugar Canto, CUICACALLI / House of Song,* and *FirstPoems*; two chapbooks, *enduring azucares* and *Hibiscus Tacos*; and a short story collection, *flesh to bone*, which won the Premio Aztlán. She and poet Dan Vera are also the co-editors of *Imaniman: Poets Writing in the Anzaldúan Borderlands*, a collection of poetry and essays. ire'ne is the recipient of a 2021 Tasajillo Writers Grant, a 2017 NALAC Fund for the Arts grant, and the final Alfredo Cisneros del Moral Award and was the fiction finalist for A Room of Her Own's 2013 Gift of Freedom award. Most recently, ire'ne was awarded the 2021 Texas Institute of Letters Shrake Award for Best Short Nonfiction. ire'ne is currently a writer-at-large for *Texas Highways* and is working on a second collection of short stories, titled *the light of your body*. Her website is irenelarasilva.wordpress.com.

Josie Méndez-Negrete, PhD, is professor emerita in Mexican American studies from the Department of Bicultural-Bilingual Studies at the University of Texas at San Antonio. Duke University Press published *Las hijas de Juan: Daughters Betrayed* as a revised edition in 2006 and reprinted it in 2010. In 2015 the University of New Mexico Press published her second book, *A Life on Hold: Living with Schizophrenia*. From 2009 to 2014, Méndez-Negrete was the lead editor of *Chicana/Latina Studies: The Journal of Mujeres Activas en Letras y Cambio Social*. She was chair of the National Association for Chicana and Chicano Studies and Mujeres Activas en Letras y Cambio

Social. The author of various articles, her most recent work, *Activist Leaders of San José, California: En sus propias voces* (2021), was published by the University of Arizona Press. She is also the publisher of Conocimientos Press, and the first publication, by Claudia D. Hernández, *Women, Mujeres, Ixoq: Revolutionary Visions*, received the 2019 International Latino Book Gold Medal award. To date, she has published nine books and is working on the tenth one.

Maria R. Palacios is a disability activist, poet, writer, artist, workshop facilitator, and professional presenter who has been passionately educating the nondisabled world about the lives, rights, and realities of disabled people for over thirty years. Through her art Maria has been a voice for the rights of disabled women, disabled immigrants, and parents with disabilities. Her work on ableism and multicultural representation of artistic advocacy is used by colleges and universities across the nation. Her work includes various genres of art, ranging from published collections of rebellious poetic storytelling to passionate spoken-word pieces and sarcastic illustrations of disability-themed cartoons aimed at calling out ableism. Maria R. Palacios is the author of several publications relating her personal experience as a disabled woman of color existing in an ableist world. María currently works for Sins Invalid, a disability-justice performance project and movement-building organization for which she has been performing since 2007. In the artistic world, María R. Palacios is known as the Goddess on Wheels.

Hector Rivera-Lopez is a Latinx clinical psychologist with more than fifty years in the field of psychology. He graduated from the University of Puerto Rico in 1970 and studied at the Wright Institute in Berkeley, California, where he was granted a PhD in clinical psychology. Dr. Rivera-Lopez focused most of his career in working with diverse Latinx communities and men's health issues. He has taught at various educational institutions in both Puerto Rico and California and is a frequent speaker at national and international conferences. He participates in a weekly telehealth program that focuses on Latinx families' health issues and a weekly men's group called Hombres Creando Lazos de Comunidad. Dr. Rivera-Lopez also is co-author of a book with three other academics, titled *Cultura y Corazón*: A Decolonial Methodology for Community Engaged Research.

Maria Angelina Soldatenko is an emeritus professor. After holding tenure-track appointments a both California State University, Northridge, and Arizona State University, she taught for twenty-three years at Pitzer College in the Chicana/o-Latina-/o Transnational Studies field group and at the Intercollegiate Department of Chicana/o Latina/o Studies at the Claremont Colleges. Her main work focused on Latina garment workers in Los Angeles. She did the first ethnographic work in a sweatshop. She published her work in journals like *Aztlán, Frontiers,* and *Cultural Studies.* Some of the work covering Chicana and Latina labor organizing has been anthologized.

Anita Tijerina Revilla is a muxerista and *jotería* activist scholar, professor, and chair of the California State University, Los Angeles, Department of Chicana(o) and Latina(o) Studies. Her research focuses on student movements and social justice education, specifically in the areas of Chicana/Latina, immigrant, feminist, and queer rights activism. Her expertise is in the areas of jotería studies, Chicanx education, Chicana/Latina feminism, and critical race and ethnic studies. Dr. Tijerina Revilla is a Harlandale High School graduate from the Southside of San Antonio. She received a bachelor's degree from Princeton University and master's degree from Teachers College, Columbia University. She earned a doctorate from the University of California, Los Angeles, graduate school of education in social sciences and comparative education with an emphasis in race and ethnic studies. She is also a visual artist who specializes in painting the muxerista and queer community.

Mónica Torreiro-Casal comes from Spain and holds a PhD in counseling psychology from Northeastern University and a master's in marriage and family therapy with an emphasis on latino mental health from Santa Clara University. She is a trained psychologist who has worked with immigrant and diverse populations in the Netherlands and the United States. As a trained psychologist, she has worked extensively in the community and in university counseling services (working with domestic violence, addiction, LGBTQIA issues, immigrants, and school and university counseling services). She is a lecturer at the Department of Chicana/o Studies at the University of California, Davis, and she has been teaching seven undergraduate classes, on mental health, immigration and health disparities, family psychology, and qualitative research methods. She conducts research on immigration and mental health, and she mentors students on their research projects. She is the co-author with Professor Flores of the books *Chicanx and Latinx Psychology: A Decolonial Approach* (Great River Learning, 2022) and *Psychological Perspectives on Chicanx and Latinx Families* (Cognella, 2021).

Enriqueta Valdez-Curiel is a medical doctor who graduated from the University of Guadalajara, Mexico. She earned a masters in community development with a specialty in rural women's health at the University of California, Davis, and did a postdoc in reproductive health policy at the Center for International Reproductive Health Policy Research at the University of California, San Francisco. Dr. Valdez-Curiel is certified in health communication leadership by the Johns Hopkins Bloomberg School of Public Health and in behavioral impact communication by the World Health Organization and New York University. She has been a professor and researcher at the University of Guadalajara School of Medicine for twenty-two years and also works as an international consultant in the area of communication for social change.

Index

Note: Page numbers in *italics* refer to illustrative matter.